THE COMPLETE GUIDE TO
KETTLEBELL TRAINING

Allan Collins

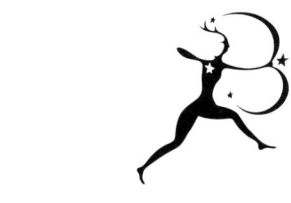

B L O O M S B U R Y

Note
Whilst every effort has been made to ensure that the content of this book is as technically accurate and as sound as possible, neither the author nor the publishers can accept responsibility for any injury or loss sustained as a result of the use of this material.

Published by Bloomsbury Publishing Plc
49–51 Bedford Square
London WC1B 3DP
www.bloomsbury.com

First edition 2011

Copyright © 2011 Allan Collins

ISBN 978 1 4081 4023 9

LIBRARIES NI	
C900234954	
Bertrams	01/03/2012
613.713	£19.99
LURGRP	

All rights reserved. No part of this publication may be reproduced in any form or by any means – graphic, electronic or mechanical, including photocopying, recording, taping or information storage and retrieval systems – without the prior permission in writing of the publishers.

Allan Collins has asserted his rights under the Copyright, Design and Patents Act, 1988, to be identified as the author of this work.

A CIP catalogue record for this book is available from the British Library.

Acknowledgements
Cover photograph © Shutterstock and Mike Harrington
All inside photographs © Mike Harrington with the exception of the following: p. 2 © Getty Images; p. 5 (top), p. 167 © Shutterstock
Designed by James Watson
Commissioned by Charlotte Croft
Edited by Rebecca Senior

This book is produced using paper that is made from wood grown in managed, sustainable forests. It is natural, renewable and recyclable. The logging and manufacturing processes conform to the environmental regulations of the country of origin.

Typeset in 10.75pt on 14pt Adobe Caslon by Saxon Graphics Ltd, Derby

Printed and bound in Spain by GraphyCems

CONTENTS

Foreword — vii

Acknowledgements — ix

Introduction — xi

PART ONE   The Basics

Chapter 1	The history of kettlebell training	2
Chapter 2	The kettlebell	4
Chapter 3	The benefits of kettlebell training	13
Chapter 4	Getting started	18
Chapter 5	Safety considerations	20
Chapter 6	Different grips and positions	23

PART TWO   The Exercises

Chapter 7	Kettlebell warm-up	34
Chapter 8	Preparation exercises	48
Chapter 9	Foundation exercises	53
Chapter 10	Exercise progressions	91

PART THREE Training Recommendations

Chapter 11 Training parameters and application   152

Chapter 12 Example training sessions   161

Chapter 13 Competitive kettlebell training   167

Glossary   168

References   170

Index   171

FOREWORD

My hope is that this book will provide you with a huge arsenal of varied and progressive kettlebell exercises with which to practice. Just as important as knowing different progressions and regressions, if not more so, is the application of these drills. Do not try to skip through the easier or more familiar variations just to try something different. Although the saying 'practice makes perfect' is commonly used, it is not correct. Only 'perfect practice' will make 'perfect', so dedicate sufficient time to train with each drill … at least 300–500 repetitions. It is only around this volume, with good technique, that your motor patterns will start to become more natural and subconscious. If you are considering becoming an elite kettlebell lifter, be aware that this will take considerable time, commonly estimated at approximately 10,000 hours of practice, which for two hours of kettlebell training a day, every day of the year, would take about 13–14 years.

Some of the variations of style will be suitable if you are looking at competing in Girevoy Sport competitions (see page 73), but that is not for everyone. Even then, try not to simply copy the technique or style of an elite lifter because you think that is the most efficient style for you – it may not be. Elite lifters have perfected their own unique style, based on what is most efficient and energy conserving for them. Only with practice and refinement will you find the style that is most suitable for you.

My best piece of advice would be to integrate this training tool alongside the other pieces of equipment in your training 'toolbox'. Fitness instructors, personal trainers or strength and conditioning coaches who rely on one training method or one piece of equipment will only limit their potential and that of their clients. I strongly advocate using dumbbells, barbells, medicine balls, unstable training tools, cables, ropes and other equipment alongside kettlebells to get the most out of them and train with variety. Use the basic human movement patterns as your template for sessions and programmes and you will find the benefits are greater and will have more carryover than trying to follow a bodybuilder-style programme.

Good health and happy training.

Allan Collins
2011

ACKNOWLEDGEMENTS

As with any significant achievement, there are always a number of people who provide support, guidance and inspiration. I would like to dedicate this book to my partner, family, friends and business partner, each of whom has helped me get to this point in my life and career. Jenny has supported me during the good and tough times, as well as being a continuing sounding board for my various ideas. My parents and sister have always supported me to do whatever made me happy, and encouraged me to thrive in an industry that does not always achieve the recognition it deserves. Without my business partner Leon, who has enlightened me to entrepreneurial flair, as well as other skills, I would never have been able to set up the education business I knew the UK market needed.

I would like to thank Charlotte Croft at Bloomsbury for her support throughout this project and the team's dedication to the development of quality education material for fitness professionals.

My last thanks goes to all of the great trainers and educators that I have learned a lot from over the years, and the students and clients I have taught and trained, who have taught me as much as I taught them, and who gave me the opportunity to try new things and pioneer different, exciting methods of training.

As with any educational material, I have tried to provide knowledge that will be true and correct for many decades, but understand that things will always evolve. My advice would be to keep an open mind and, as I do, look for the simplest, most logical answer for any question you may have – it is usually the correct one.

Enjoy your training, listen to your body and good health.

INTRODUCTION

Kettlebell training has developed over the last number of years into one of the most popular forms of training within the fitness industry. What started out as a little used, relatively unknown piece of equipment, utilised by a select few underground trainers in the 1990s has, during the last 10 years, become an essential tool in many methodologies of training, and is now sold by virtually all retailers of fitness equipment.

So what makes the kettlebell so unique? What makes it so much better than a barbell, a dumbbell, a medicine ball, or any of the other training tools? Well, in answer to that question, it is not better, just different. Good trainers will never limit themselves to using a single tool. However, the kettlebell is a very versatile tool, and so if it can be used for a variety of different exercises, working different muscles across a range of human movement patterns, we should then try to utilise it as much as possible, where appropriate. As with all pieces of equipment and exercises, the kettlebell will be suitable for some with certain goals and starting points and unsuitable for others.

The kettlebell can be used to improve grip strength and endurance, teach a correct lifting technique and develop strength and endurance in the hamstrings, gluteals and back muscles. It will help improve coordination and proprioception, is commonly used as a preferred tool for fat loss, and can even give its users improvements in aerobic and anaerobic fitness. It is used by many athletes from the rugby, mixed martial arts (MMA), football and tennis worlds, as well as armed forces across the world, police, fire service and SWAT teams. It can be used indoors or outdoors and is durable, with the potential to last for decades.

The Complete Guide to Kettlebell Training has been written to not only describe a huge variety of exercise techniques, progressions, regressions and variations, but also to give you the knowledge and tools to be able to correctly apply these techniques. Rather than telling you this style or that style is the only way to perform a certain drill, I believe it is better to give the reader the key information about how to safely perform a drill and give you options to try to find the most efficient way, for you, to perform these tasks.

I have taught hundreds of fitness instructors and personal trainers over the many years I have been a part of the fitness industry. In that time I have drawn upon my knowledge of and experience in traditional strength and conditioning, biomechanical analysis and modern concepts of functional and primal human movement training to give you the best advice in relation to kettlebell training and its applications.

1

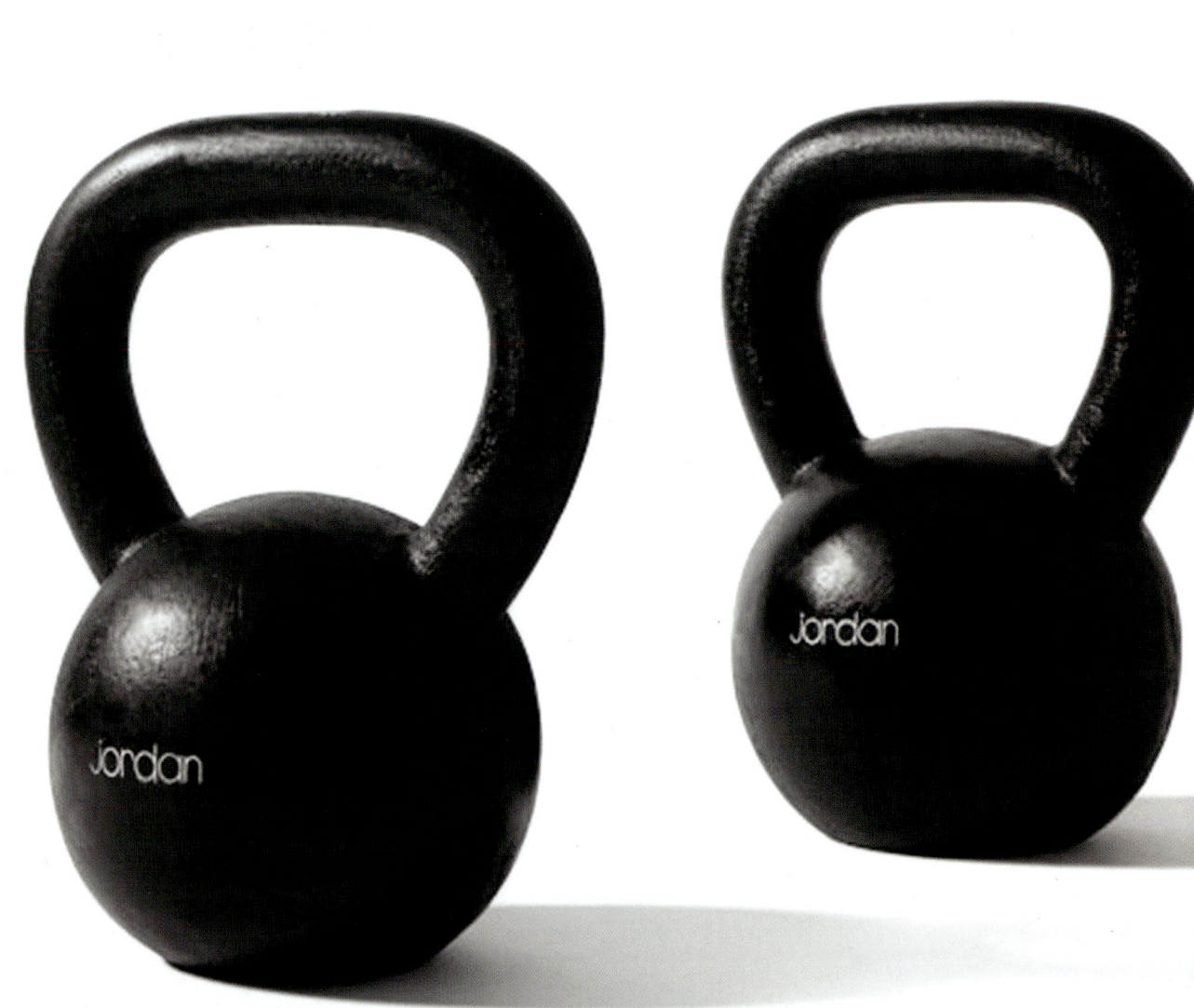

PART ONE

THE BASICS

THE HISTORY OF KETTLEBELL TRAINING

The kettlebell, or *girya* as it is known in Russia, is a cast iron weight which looks somewhat like a cannonball with a handle. The kettlebell differs from a dumbbell in that a dumbbell has a single handle with weights, or load, at both ends, while the kettlebell has a single load and a handle of some description coming off it.

Different types of weights with handles have been seen in the historical records of many different countries, including Greece, Russia, Scotland and others. Although there is much debate about which country or individual was the first to utilise kettlebells, we do know that strongmen and other advocates of physical culture have used them for well over a hundred years. Although the kettlebell has had a recent revival, it is certainly not a new training tool, but it can probably best be described as somewhat of a forgotten tool.

VICTORIAN STRONGMEN

Eugen Sandow (see figure 1.1) was one of the most reputable strongman-bodybuilders in Victorian times and was a personal trainer to many famous people, including British royalty. A bronze statue of Sandow has been presented to the winner of the Mr Olympia contest since 1977 in recognition of his status and achievements in the world of bodybuilding. The photo shows the main tools used by Sandow to develop strength and his physique – heavy thick barbells and dumbbells, ropes and, by his feet, two kettlebells.

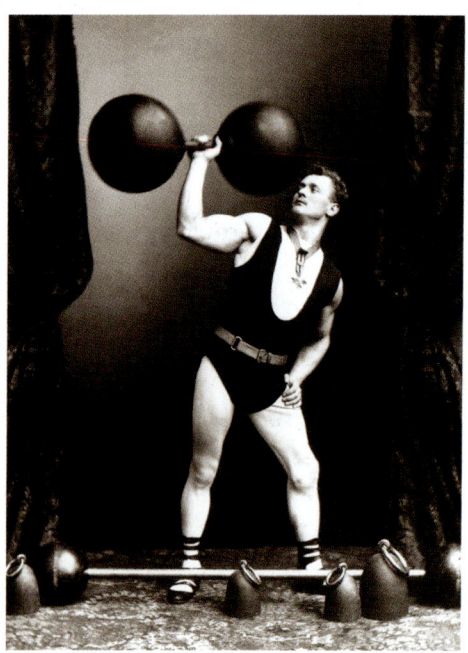

Figure 1.1 Eugen Sandow

Although not recruited as extensively for swings and snatches as modern kettlebells are today, Victorian strongmen used the kettlebell in a traditional feat of strength known as the 'two-hands anyhow'. In this exercise, the strongman raised a dumbbell or barbell above his head by whatever method he desired, then he bent down and picked up a second weight, commonly a kettlebell, curled it to his shoulder and then stood up and pressed or jerked the weight above his head as well! The kettlebell was commonly used as the second weight to be lifted because of its handled design and the fact that it was slightly higher off the ground than the dumbbell, making it slightly easier to lift.

While vintage-style strongman training was gradually becoming less popular through the 1900s, the Russians were embracing the kettlebell as a major training tool for swinging, lifting, pressing, throwing and juggling.

RECENT DEVELOPMENTS

In the 1990s, several kettlebell pioneers, such as Pavel Tsatsouline, brought the concept of kettlebell training to the United States where it began to flourish and expand before spreading to other countries. Pavel ran Russian Kettlebell Certification (RKC) courses throughout the world and taught what is now commonly referred to as the 'hard style' of kettlebell training.

Since the 1980s there has also been an influx of kettlebell competitions, initially in Russia and now across a number of countries. The goal in Olympic weightlifting is to achieve maximal weight, i.e. the amount of weight/load that can be lifted in a single repetition. However, kettlebell events differ in that they are designed to test strength-endurance and power-endurance by having the lifters complete as many repetitions within a 10-minute period as they can. Kettlebell sport, or Girevoy Sport (GS), has become more and more popular with elite lifters, such as Valery Fedorenko, and the delivery of GS or fluid-style courses and training has flourished.

Functional training can be defined as performing exercises that will improve your ability or efficiency to perform your daily tasks, your occupation or your sport, or that will improve your resilience to injury. As both trainers and clients embrace the concept of functional training to reduce the risk of injury and help improve performance when undertaking daily tasks or aiming for athletic success, different training tools have been evaluated for their effectiveness in meeting these goals. Barbells, dumbbells, bodyweight and cables have been used for some time to meet the needs of functional training. Today, kettlebells have resurfaced as a viable alternative, as many embrace the simplicity and enjoyment of lifting and moving the weights that Victorian strongmen viewed as a critical part of physical culture. Kettlebells are becoming a staple piece of training equipment and can now be found in most health clubs, fitness centres and gyms, alongside the cardiovascular and fixed path machines and the traditional free weights equipment.

// THE KETTLEBELL 2

Ten years ago, there were only a couple of different types of kettlebell available to buy, and from very few distributors. However, over the last few years there has been a huge increase in the popularity of kettlebell training and consequently there is now a huge variety of kettlebells available for the trainer or client to purchase. See table 2.1 for further information on the various categories and weights available.

TYPES OF KETTLEBELL

There are two main categories of kettlebell type, what I describe as fitness kettlebells and competition kettlebells.

COMPETITION KETTLEBELLS

These kettlebells meet certain dimension requirements, set out by the organisations that run official kettlebell competitions throughout the world. In international terms, the World Kettlebell Club (WKC), the International Union of Kettlebell Lifting (IUKL) and the IGSF (International Girya Sport Federation) are the most prominent ones. Competition kettlebells are a uniform size, whether the bell weighs 8kg or 40kg, which means that when a client is learning a technique the kettlebell size remains standard as they start to progress through the different weights. Competition bells can be of benefit to those looking to compete in kettlebell lifting, as every repetition of a drill is performed in exactly the same way, whether the bell is heavy or light.

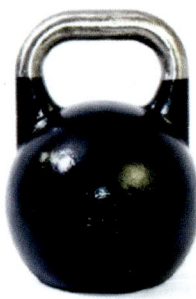

Figure 2.1 A competition kettlebell

FITNESS KETTLEBELLS

With fitness kettlebells the size of the bell increases in proportion to the weight, meaning that techniques for exercises such as the clean or snatch may need to be altered slightly to accommodate the changes in the dimensions of the bell.

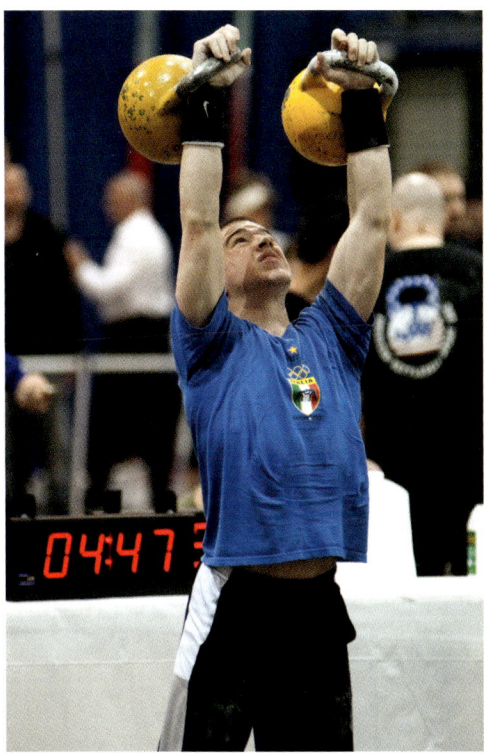

Figure 2.2 Competition kettlebells in use

Fitness-style kettlebells are classified as any other type of kettlebell that doesn't meet competition requirements. They are usually made from cast iron (unlike the steel competition version), and are sometimes coated with neoprene, vinyl, rubber or plastic.

Many fitness centres and health clubs prefer the coloured varieties, as they are colour-coded for different weights. It has also been said that cast iron bells do not attract female members as they are too intimidating. From my perspective, this view seems rather patronising towards women, but if having colourful neoprene-coated bells gets more clients to try them, then this can be taken as a positive.

A newer type of fitness-style kettlebell is the chrome-handled rubber version. Some prefer these bells as they have a smooth handle, unlike the slightly grainy texture of the cast iron handles. However, caution should be taken when the hands get sweaty as the grip can be lost. Many clients use training gloves with these bells to reduce this risk.

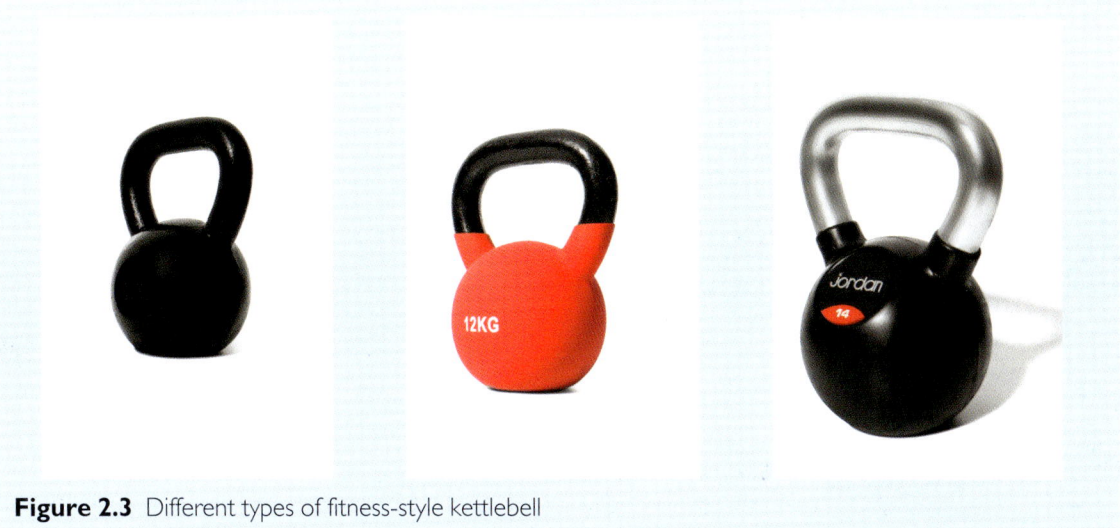

Figure 2.3 Different types of fitness-style kettlebell

> **Rusting**
> Exposing steel and cast iron kettlebells to rain and air may cause them to rust, so be careful about leaving your kettlebells outside and, as much as possible, clean and dry them after each use.

KETTLEBELL WEIGHTS

Kettlebells are usually available in weights from 4kg (9lb) up to 40kg (88lb). Kettlebells in the UK show weight in kilograms, while in the US the weight of the bells is shown in pounds. Most companies offer kettlebells in increments of 4kg (see table 2.1), although some manufacturers have started offering increments of 2kg. This is particularly useful for making smaller incremental increases in load. For example, you might be using an 8kg bell for overhead pressing and you need to go up a weight for continued overload; progressing to a 12kg bell would be an increase of 50 per cent on your previous weight, which is way above the recommended increase in load.

As you can see in table 2.1, kettlebells have previously been referred to in terms of poods. A pood is a unit of mass equal to approximately 16.38kg (36.11lb), and it was used in Russia and several other Eastern European countries to describe weight. Today, this is an outdated term but it is still used to describe the weight with modern kettlebells, as a tradition more than a necessity of it being an exact weight. Kettlebells are therefore sometimes referred to in multiples or fractions of 16kg. For example, a 32kg kettlebell is two poods.

Table 2.1 Converting traditional poods to kilograms/pounds

Poods	Kgs	Lbs
0.25	4	9
0.50	8	18
0.75	12	27
1.00	16	36
1.25	20	45
1.50	24	54
1.75	28	63
2.00	32	72
2.50	40	90
3.00	48	106

It is recommended that an average male start with a 16kg (36lb) bell and an average female start with a 12kg (27lb) bell. These 'standard' recommendations would be applicable for average size, strength and fitness levels, and for the majority of exercises, but one should also take into account a number of factors:

- **Previous training history**: For an individual who has undertaken good quality strength training for a period of at least 1–2 years, a heavier starting bell may be more suitable, although not always. Females particularly may be able to use a 16kg bell or heavier if they have undertaken training programmes that have included exercises such as barbell deadlifts, squats, pull-ups or the barbell Olympic lifts (clean, snatch, jerk).
- **Kettlebell exercise**: Different exercises require slight variation in the load (or weight of bell) that you use. You wouldn't expect to deadlift, bench press and bicep curl the same weight, and the same is true with kettlebells. You should lift the heaviest weights when performing the clean, jerk and the two hand swing. The Turkish get-up and the overhead squat often requires a lighter weight. If you can snatch a 16kg bell, you will need a heavier weight when doing your two hand swings.
- **Duration of the set**: The longer the set is, the more the emphasis turns from strength and power to strength-endurance and power-endurance. Longer sets, with more repetitions, usually require a lighter weight.
- **Quality of technique**: Do not compromise the quality of the exercise technique at any time for any reason. If the technique is not what it should be, then the load is usually lowered to assist skill acquisition. Sometimes, however, trainers may find that too light a weight also makes it difficult to learn the correct technique. Is your kettlebell flying too high during a swing? Use a heavier bell. Is it banging hard on your forearm when you snatch an 8kg bell? Try a heavier bell.
- **Competition**: Males use anything from two 12kg bells up to two 32kg bells for competitions, whereas females use anything from 8kg up to 24kg kettlebells.

When selecting kettlebell weights for your foundation drills, there may be some variations depending on the exercise. For this reason it is usually best to get a small set of various weights, which allows for these differences (see table 2.2).

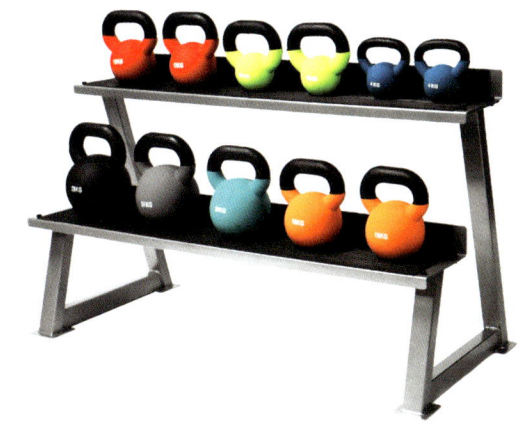

Figure 2.4 A rack of fitness-style kettlebells

Table 2.2 Suggested kettlebell set for various groups	
Description	Ideal kettlebell set
Beginner female	8kg, 12kg, 16kg
Beginner male	12kg, 16kg, 20kg
Advanced	Two of 12kg, 16kg, 20kg, 28kg, 32kg

ANATOMY OF A BELL

It is important to know the basic terms used to describe the different parts of the kettlebell. This will help when you get to the exercise variations later in the book, but it is also useful to know when you are considering which kettlebell brand to purchase.

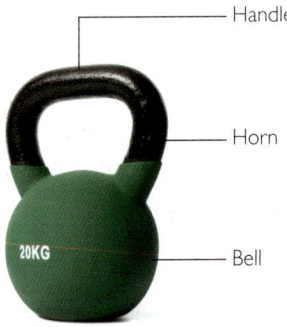

Figure 2.5 The kettlebell anatomy

1. The 'bell' part of the kettlebell is usually round in shape and is the part that looks like a cannonball. The bell is the area where the majority of the weight is housed.
2. The 'handle' is the horizontal section above the bell, which can be straight or slightly curved, and is held by the user with either one or two hands.
3. The two 'horns' connect the 'handle' to the 'bell' and again may be straight, slightly curved, vertical or at a slight angle.

Kettlebell horns
Some kettlebells have a really long handle and long horns at almost 45 degrees, while others have really short horns with the handle close to the bell.

CHOOSING A KETTLEBELL BY DESIGN

So what design factors should be considered when choosing a kettlebell? Choosing a well designed bell will make it easier to learn the correct positions and techniques for many of the drills, while a poorly designed bell will make it virtually impossible to acquire the correct skills for the clean, press, squat, snatch, Turkish get-up and variations of these. Consider the handle length, horn length, the size of the handle and handle texture when choosing a kettlebell.

Handle length
It is preferable that the handle length isn't too long, since a long handle makes it very difficult and uncomfortable when performing cleans and snatches. Although it may not make as big a difference during exercises like the two hand swing, it is better not to choose a bell that is only good for a few drills. You want to be able to perform lots of different exercises with your chosen bell.

You should be able to comfortably hold the handle with one hand, with a very slight gap between the little finger and the end of the handle. This length of handle is ideal for cleans, snatches, jerks and presses. When holding the handle with two hands, you should find that the little fingers and maybe the ring fingers do not really grip the handle. If you can get both hands fully on the handle, then it is too long.

Size of handle

Choose a handle that is a comfortable diameter for the size of your hand. Competition kettlebells have a uniform handle size for all weights, whereas some of the fitness-style kettlebells have slightly thicker handles for the heavier weights of 16kg or 20kg upwards and slightly thinner for 12kg and below.

Thick handles, although great for hand and forearm strength and endurance improvements with drills like the farmer's walk, cause your forearm muscles to fatigue too quickly during repetitive swings or snatches and can be counterproductive.

Handle texture

A cast iron handle should have a slightly grainy texture to it, allowing the user to get a good grip when performing certain drills. The kettlebell doesn't need to be gripped rigidly for most drills, for example in the swing and snatch, so this texture prevents the handle from slipping out of a loose grip.

Some kettlebell designs have a very prominent ridge on the underside of the handle. This is somewhat inconsequential for certain exercises, like the press, squat and swing. However, for two of the key drills – the clean and the snatch – the handle has to rotate through 180 degrees in a loosely held grip, and the ridge can cause excessive discomfort, which can lead to blisters and calluses on the hands.

There are some kettlebells with knurling (the crisscross effect that is seen on barbells and dumbbells), but you should avoid these. For drills where the kettlebell is relatively static, such as a press or windmill or Turkish get-up, the knurling isn't an issue. However, for all dynamic drills, such as swings, cleans, snatches, etc., it is critical that the handle rotates within the palm. The grainy surface found on most kettlebells is fine in this instance, but knurling is designed to grip and it will rip the skin from your hand. You can perform a snatch or clean with a knurl-handled Olympic bar as the bar doesn't spin within the grip, but on the bearings instead. Thus, you avoid the potential discomfort.

Horn length

The horns connect the handle to the bell and dictate the gap between the two. This is important since if this gap is too small it makes it virtually impossible to achieve correct technique with many common drills, such as the snatch, press, Turkish get-up and clean. This is because when holding a bell with a short horn in these drills it will end up

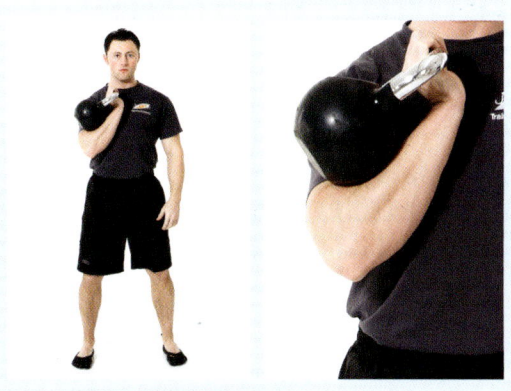

Figure 2.6 A bell with a short horn can lead to a subconscious cocking of the wrist.

sitting between, or near, the condyles (bony prominences) of the wrist/forearm.

This is quite uncomfortable, so individuals may subconsciously cock their wrist (see figure 2.6) into an extended or hyper-extended position so that the bell sits lower on the forearm with more muscle 'cushioning'. With the wrist in a straight position, which is referred to as the 'rack position', the bell part of the kettlebell should sit more on the fleshy part of the forearm just below the wrist.

> ### Testing your kettlebell
> Some of the more angular-shaped horns are particularly bad for encouraging the user to have the bell sit on the forearm by cocking their wrist. Therefore, it is recommended that you try a few repetitions of exercises such as the clean or snatch to determine wrist comfort before purchasing a kettlebell. If the handle is too long, then the horns are usually quite long and stick out at quite an angle, making it easier for you to recognise.

KETTLEBELL ATTACHMENTS AND ADDITIONAL TRAINING AIDS

There are some real innovators in the field of kettlebell attachments and additional training aids. Anthony DiLuglio, founder of the Kettlebell Gyms and Art of Strength™ training facilities in the United States, has come up with, among others, two great additions to the standard kettlebell: the kettlebell buddy and the kettlebell leash.

THE KETTLEBELL BUDDY

The Kettlebell Buddy™ is a 2kg weight that is screwed into the base of the Art of Strength™ kettlebells providing a small incremental increase in the load, which is particularly helpful when using the lighter kettlebells and you want to get only a slight increase. Going from an 8kg bell to a 12kg bell is an increase of 50 per cent in weight, which is far too much progression in relation to the standard recommendations. Imagine if somebody told you to go from your dumbbell presses with two x 20kg to two x 30kg dumbbells … it's likely you wouldn't be able to! This is what makes the Kettlebell Buddy™ unique and ultimately a very useful piece of kit. Some manufacturers do supply kettlebells in the intermediate ranges (6kg, 10kg, 14kg), but these are few and far between, which is another reason why the Kettlebell Buddy™ is so useful.

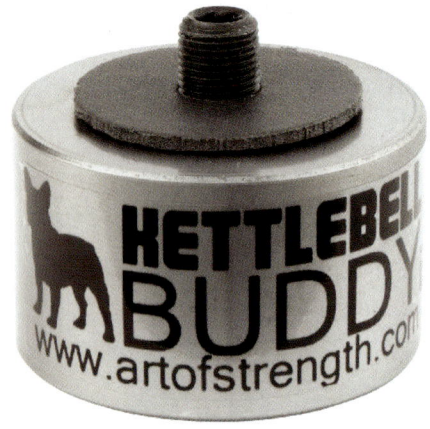

Figure 2.7 The Kettlebell Buddy™

THE KETTLEBELL LEASH

The Kettlebell Leash™ is a chain that also attaches to the base of the Art of Strength™ kettlebells. Some may see this and think 'what's the point of that?' However, when you actually get to use the kettlebell leash, you begin to appreciate the benefits. Not only does it provide an incremental increase in load but, more importantly, it increases resistance from the dragging effect of the chain on the floor. This is really effective for training and improving technique and in particular it stimulates great activation of the glutes and hamstrings muscles. It can also be used as a method of 'progressive resistance' where the load increases during the concentric (lifting) phase of the exercise, such as when performing the windmill or overhead press. This will provide a different type of loading to many standard exercises, allowing for continued strength improvements. The progressive resistance method is becoming very popular with those who use many standard resistance tools, such as the Olympic bar and EZ bar, to provide a new stimulus to the body for continued fitness adaptations.

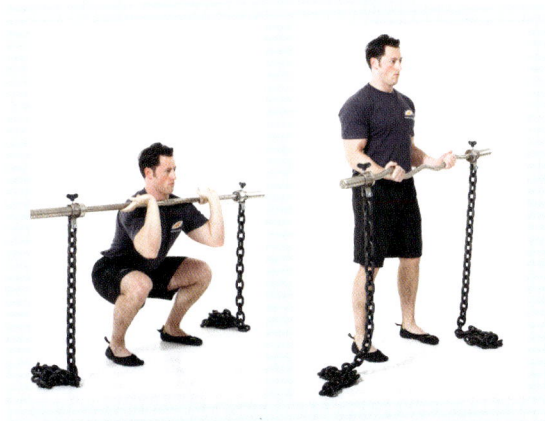

Figure 2.9 Examples of progressive resistance

USING A TOWEL

A towel can be used with some kettlebell drills. The towel is fed through the handle and gripped in either one or both hands for swings. This stimulates the muscles used for gripping in the hand and forearm, as well as taking the load further from the body, increasing the lever arm and providing more overload for the lifting muscles of the posterior chain (hamstrings, glutes, lower back) for improved

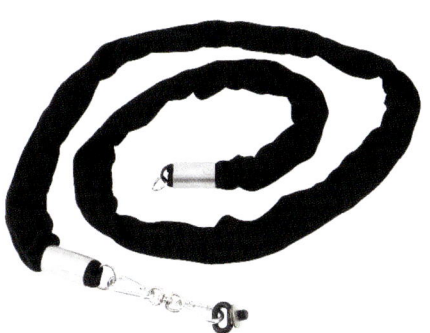

Figure 2.8 The kettlebell leash

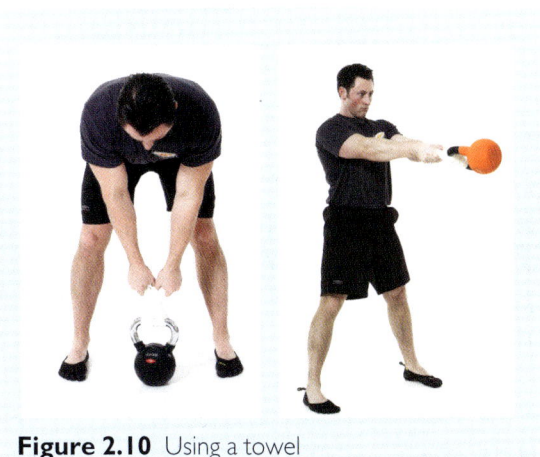

Figure 2.10 Using a towel

strength and for back health. This same towel grip can also be used as a variation for common drills such as the bicep curl or hammer curl.

USING A FIT BAR

The fit bar (sometimes called the strength bar or body bar) is a weighted bar, commonly found in most studios around the world. The fit bar can be used as a variation, regression or progression for many of the foundation kettlebell drills, from the windmill, overhead squat and side press to the two hands anyhow. Although not great for the kettlebell swings, it can be a great a resource for personal trainers and other fitness professionals to use when there are more attendees in a group kettlebell training class than actual kettlebells.

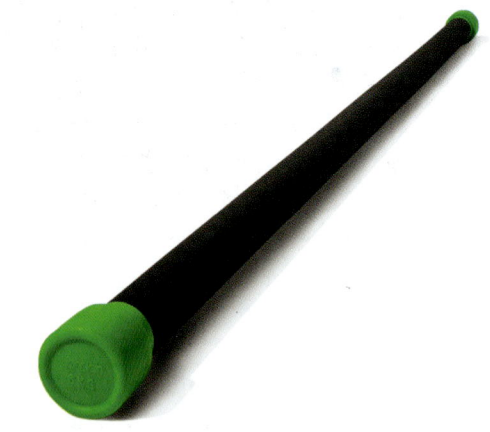

Figure 2.11 Using a fit bar as an alternative to a kettlebell for some of the common drills

THE BENEFITS OF KETTLEBELL TRAINING

3

Kettlebells are an excellent addition to the arsenal of different tools that a trainer can use for their clients. The kettlebell can be used as an alternative to many other types of free weights, such as the dumbbell, as well as facilitating cardiovascular adaptations. They are more comfortable than dumbbells for many exercises, such as the overhead press and Turkish get-up, because of the way they sit on the forearm. However, they are most beneficial over other freeweights for dynamic resistance training because of their design and the fact that the bell will rotate around the handle. Dynamic resistance training would include exercises such as the swing, the (swing) snatch and the (swing) clean – dynamic, rhythmical resistance exercises that are continuous and overload the cardio-respiratory system as much as the muscular system.

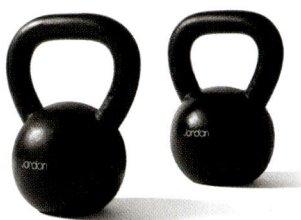

Figure 3.1 Kettlebells can be used to develop cardiovascular fitness.

FREE WEIGHTS

The kettlebell is classified as a free weight, alongside barbells, plates, dumbbells, medicine balls, powerbags and any other type of weight that is unrestricted. Free weights have been, and always will be, a great tool for improving fitness, since lifting, throwing, dragging and all other basic human patterns that we have undertaken throughout history have almost always involved an external weight. Since the time of the Ancient Greeks and Romans, structured exercise has been a popular method of improving human performance (initially to develop combat skills) and these methods have always made use of different types of free weights. Soldiers used spears, hammers, shields and nets to practise fighting techniques and develop task-specific fitness. Later, Victorian strongmen used barbells, kettlebells, dumbbells, cables, bodyweight drills (such as pull-ups) and wrestling. In the 1960s the industry moved away from free weights towards the fixed path era. However, today, functional training and unconventional or caveman-style training, such as tyre flipping or sledge hammer slams, is becoming popular again and we are starting to move full circle and embrace the tools and training of previous generations.

The benefits of free weight training

Free weight strength and conditioning exercises are unsupported, involve a greater use of core and other stabiliser muscles, and have more carryover to other sports and everyday life. Prolonged overemphasis of fixed path training may cause overuse issues and development of faulty movement patterns.

Figure 3.2 The lift pattern – kettlebell swing or barbell deadlift

HUMAN MOVEMENT PATTERNS

Humans have undertaken particular movement patterns for thousands of years, and we should incorporate these same patterns into our structured exercise programme to best improve performance.

Kettlebells can be used to train a variety of primal human movement patterns, in particular the lift, press and pull patterns (see table 3.1).

This book demonstrates a range of kettlebell exercises that fit into the major movement patterns and allow for the full spectrum of human movements to be improved within a training programme (see chapter 12, in particular the first table, for further information on which exercises you can incorporate into your training programme to work specific movement patterns).

Table 3.1	Human movement patterns
Pattern type	Description
Squat	A quadriceps-dominant exercise, involving a sitting action
Lift	A hip extensor or hamstring-dominant exercise, where the body bends forward
Press	Involving the chest, shoulders and triceps, where the body is pushed away from an object or an object pushed away from the body
Pull	Involving the back, shoulders and biceps, where the body is pulled towards an object or an object pulled towards the body
Rotation	Any twisting motion of the body, whether horizontal, diagonally upwards or diagonally downwards
Smash	A flexion motion (bending motion) of the body, used to accelerate an object forwards or downwards
Moving or carrying load	Moving weight from one position to another by carrying, dragging or any other means
Gait and locomotion	Moving the body from one place to another across varying environments. Includes walking, running, swimming and crawling

METABOLIC ACCELERATION

Kettlebells are always strongly advocated as being particularly effective for increasing metabolism and initiating positive changes in body composition. Farrar, Mayhew & Koch (2010) found that 'Continuous kettlebell swings can impart a metabolic challenge of sufficient intensity to increase VO_2max'. The tests compared the results of 12 minutes of swings with a 16kg bell to a VO_2max graded exercise test and concluded that the kettlebell swings resulted in a significantly higher heart rate.

Therefore, training at a sufficient intensity with kettlebells may initiate beneficial changes in metabolic rate, resulting in maintenance of lean muscle mass and a decrease in body fat. A significant increase in lean body mass (hypertrophy) can be achieved with kettlebell training, but is less likely and would require specific training parameters of load, reps, tempo and volume. Dumbbells, barbells and fixed path machines would be tools more suited to bodybuilding (hypertrophy) than kettlebells.

CARDIOVASCULAR BENEFITS

As shown previously, the correct application of training parameters in kettlebell conditioning can cause a significant impact on the cardiovascular system, which over a period of time may result in an increase in aerobic and anaerobic fitness.

Tabata et al (1996) looked at whether steady state or high intensity intermittent training was more efficient at improving aerobic or anaerobic fitness. The study assessed two different methods of training for six weeks, 'moderate-intensity steady state' and 'high-intensity intermittent' training. First, subjects undertook 60 minutes of moderate-intensity endurance training (intensity: 70 per cent of maximal oxygen uptake (VO_2max)) for five days/week. Results showed that the anaerobic capacity did not increase significantly, while VO_2max increased.

The high-intensity intermittent training consisted of intermittent training exercise five times per week for six weeks, of 7–8 sets of 20-second exercises at an intensity of about 170 per cent of VO_2max with a 10-second rest between each bout. After the training period, VO_2max increased by 7ml.kg-1.min-1, while the anaerobic capacity increased by 28 per cent. In conclusion, this study showed that moderate-intensity aerobic training that improves the maximal aerobic power does not change anaerobic capacity and that adequate high-intensity intermittent training may improve both anaerobic and aerobic energy supplying systems significantly, probably through imposing intensive stimuli on both systems. Although their study used a cycle ergometer, their protocol has been adapted for use with other forms of exercise. If the exerciser can reach an equivalent intensity to 170 per cent of VO_2max (translation = working really hard!) for 8 x 20 seconds with a 10-second recovery period between bouts, then similar improvements in aerobic and anaerobic fitness should be feasible.

STRENGTH ENDURANCE AND POWER ENDURANCE

Because of the common training parameters used, e.g. high repetitions, longer time-under-tension (the duration of the set or how long the muscle group is under tension), individuals undertaking kettlebell training are more likely to see improvements in their ability to produce sub-maximal forces over a prolonged period of time (strength endurance and power endurance), rather than dramatic improvements in absolute strength or power. This is not to say that individuals won't see any improvements in strength or power, because many will, but this is usually limited to those starting the training protocols who are further away from their genetic potential. It also depends greatly on the type of training applied; if an individual undertakes lots of high-load, low-rep sets, with moderate to high volume, then improvements in strength and power may well be seen.

CREATING AN EFFICIENT LINK BETWEEN UPPER AND LOWER TORSO

Many of the foundation drills, such as the two hand swing, one hand swing, snatch and clean, should improve coordination between the lower body and the upper body when performed correctly. For example, as an individual swings the kettlebell between their legs, they load the lifting muscles (hamstrings, glutes, lats) as they flex at the hips into a bent-over position. The individual should then contract the loaded muscles, bringing the hips forward, which creates momentum and force. This force should then be transferred through the core muscles to the shoulders and arms, and eventually to the handle of the kettlebell, which causes the bell to rise in an arc motion.

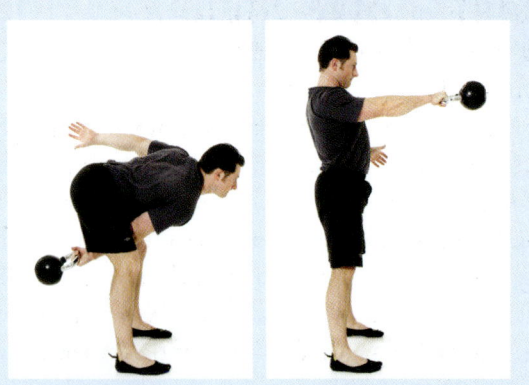

Figure 3.3 The core creates an efficient link between the hip muscles and the kettlebell

The more efficient the transfer, the more force can be generated and the more weight can be lifted or more repetitions undertaken. When there is an inefficient transfer of force, energy is lost and wasted and the resulting performance is poor. This is equivalent to someone who has great leg strength but scores poorly at vertical jump tests. The leg strength and power must be able to link in with, and be transferred through, the core and upper torso to properly show itself. We commonly see this inefficiency with certain swing techniques. Some individuals actually push the bell off the hips during the hip extension, or straightening phase. This negates the transfer of force through the core and arms and helps to 'hide' inefficiency traits which would otherwise be evident. Individuals are usually unaware of these technique adaptations, as the body simply seeks to find the easiest way to get the task done.

GRIP AND FOREARM STRENGTH AND ENDURANCE

Kettlebells can be used to improve the strength and endurance of the gripping muscles of the hand, wrist and forearm. However, this must be applied through use of very specific drills. Simply undertaken swings, cleans and snatches won't probably result in any significant improvements in grip performance. This is because the grip overload required to swing, clean or snatch a kettlebell is actually quite low. Many individuals can demonstrate these exercises holding the bell with only one or two fingers. Therefore, certain drills should be included within the training programme to increase grip strength and endurance:

- The farmer's walk (exercise 110, page 146)
- The bottoms up clean or press (exercise 99, page 138)
- The fingertip press (exercise 82, page 127)
- Hammer curls (exercise 113, page 148)
- The plank press-up or rows on two kettlebells (exercises 101 and 102, pages 139 and 141)

MENTAL FOCUS UNDER PHYSICAL STRESS

Kettlebell training can provide excellent benefits for any individual involved in combat sports, like mixed martial arts (MMA) or rugby, or those in the armed forces. Imagine an MMA fighter who has been punching and kicking intensively for two five-minute rounds, and then finds himself having to execute a complex grappling or Jiu Jitsu move. Or the soldier that has to sprint 400 yards, stop and then fire accurately at the enemy. In both instances, the ability to focus on a skills-based task when fatigued can mean the difference between success and failure. If that individual trains with multiple snatch sets, for example, after two minutes of intensive training, they must still remain focused to ensure that every repetition they make displays an effective and efficient technique of lifting, pulling and punching. This is the only way they will correctly execute the drill and be able to continue the set.

GETTING STARTED

EFFICIENCY IN KETTLEBELL TRAINING

This is written with kettlebells in mind, but the importance of efficiency of movement is by no means restricted to exercising with kettlebells. Indeed, the goal of structured exercise is to improve human efficiency; to make movements or tasks more fluid and easy with less cognitive effort and expending less energy. Whether this makes a person's job easier or improves athletic performance, it all comes down to one factor: efficiency. While trying to improve your efficiency during kettlebell exercises, remember the following key points:

THE GOLDILOCKS PRINCIPLE

We are all aware of the Goldilocks fable – a bed not too hard, not too soft … ahhh, just right! This principle works well for kettlebell training. If you need to produce sufficient force to swing a 16kg bell up to shoulder height, then you should use as little energy as possible to get the bell to that height. If the kettlebell goes above the head, then too much energy is being used; the recommendation in this case would be to use a heavier bell or produce less force.

DON'T WASTE ENERGY MAKING NOISE

Many kettlebell trainers who teach clients or run courses in kettlebell training really focus on getting their clients to make 'tchhhh'-like noises when undertaking the lift part of exercises like the swing, because they believe it ensures that clients do not hold their breath and will help teach them to maintain abdominal tension. If your style naturally evolves to make these noises, that's fine. If you find that focusing on the forced exhalation during this phase and making this noise helps with your technique, then, again, please do it. However, don't just copy your trainer's style because you think that's the most efficient way of doing it. It may be most efficient for them, but not necessarily for you.

PRACTISE BECOMING EFFICIENT

Practice develops your motor patterns, meaning your technique feels more natural, takes less conscious effort and gradually becomes the method in which your body completes that task. If you practise with good technique, then that technique will become permanent. If you practise being inefficient, then that will become permanent. Know the difference between style and technique and find out how you can be most efficient within the confines of good technique.

NOBODY LIKES A COPYCAT

Don't copy another style. Head up or head aligned while swinging? Breathe out going up or coming down? Keep the legs stiff or bend the knees? There are arguments for all of these variations in style. For example, keeping your head up can help engage the posterior chain and keep your chest up, helping you to maintain a good back position. But it may lead to shortening of certain neck muscles. Keeping your head aligned with your spine prevents this, but many clients can feel dizzy and some may round their back as a result, losing a safe and effective spinal position. Therefore, don't just copy an elite kettlebell lifter, who has developed his/her style over many years, because it may do you more harm than good in the long run. You must develop a style that works safely and efficiently for you alone.

DON'T GRIP THE KETTLEBELL TOO HARD

Kettlebells can be used to improve grip strength and endurance with certain drills, but you don't need to grip them maximally on every rep on every drill. Apply the Goldilocks principle – only grip it as hard as you need to avoid letting go – any more is simply a waste of energy.

COMPETITIONS ARE THE EPITOME OF EFFICIENCY

Many people have really embraced kettlebell training and kettlebell competitions are becoming more and more popular. There is a real difference between fitness training using kettlebells and competitive kettlebell lifting. For example, a client doing three sets of 12 reps of the snatch will want to expend as much energy as possible to help reach their fat loss goals. The competitive kettlebell lifter, on the other hand, has to snatch that bell for 10 minutes; they want to expend as little energy as possible to get the bell from between their legs to above their head. The more energy they save, the more reps they can do, or the quicker they maintain their tempo of snatches per minute. Energy saving is the key to competitive kettlebell lifting. Watch how different elite lifters position themselves to conserve energy – some of the styles may look a little odd, but don't dismiss them before first watching the huge volumes of weight they are able to lift in a 10-minute period.

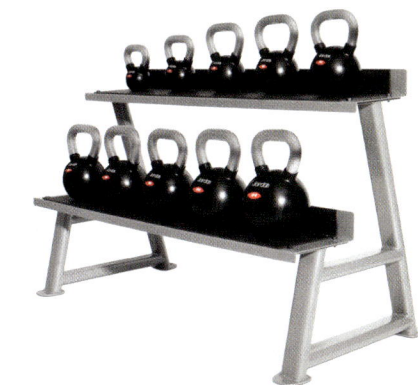

Figure 4.1 Develop your own style when using kettlebells

SAFETY CONSIDERATIONS 5

Safety is always paramount with any type of structured exercise and, because of the inherent dynamic or ballistic nature of many of the drills, training with kettlebells should always be taken seriously.

BEFORE YOU START

Consider the following safety aspects before you begin your training session:

- Check with your medical practitioner prior to commencement of kettlebell training as it can be taxing on the cardio-respiratory and musculoskeletal systems. You should therefore discuss any concerns you have regarding your health with a medical professional before beginning a new training programme.
- Ensure there is sufficient space in front, behind and to the side of you for all of the kettlebell drills you are going to undertake.
- Wear flat, supportive training shoes, such as Nike Free (see figure 5.1) or Vibram® Five Fingers (see figure 5.2). Some individuals may wish to wear Olympic weightlifting shoes, especially during competitions, to provide more support for the feet and ankles. Some fitness trainers are strong advocates of training barefoot, and while I agree with barefoot training, both with and without weights, this doesn't need to be done all the time and is dependent upon the individual fitness club's rules on footwear and hygiene.
- Wear appropriate training attire that allows you to move freely and fully, as many of the kettlebell drills require a dynamic and substantial range of movement.
- Ensure that there is enough space between you and anyone else before training, and avoid training in a thoroughfare when training in a public environment.
- Make sure the kettlebells are clean and dry to ensure a safe grip.
- Choose an appropriate training surface, such as a matted area. Think: if you drop the kettlebell, which you may have to do for safety, would the surface be damaged?
- Make sure you undertake an appropriate and thorough warm-up every session.

DURING TRAINING

As you get your training under way, keep the following safety aspects in mind as you exercise:

- Be mindful of the training environment and be aware that people may absent-mindedly walk into your training space.
- Make sure that kettlebells are placed safely between sets so as not to create a trip or fall hazard for yourself or others (see figure 5.3).
- If you lose control of your kettlebell, stop the drill immediately. If you are undertaking certain drills, such as the advanced juggling techniques, it may be safer to release/drop the kettlebell if you lose control, rather than trying to catch it, as this could injure your fingers, back or foot/leg if it hits you. Always use an appropriate surface for this type of training and be aware of the inherent risks.
- If your hands tingle or hurt during training, then stop, prior to them blistering or tearing.
- Focus on correct teaching/safety points on every rep, set and session.
- Don't practise poor technique due to fatigue or sore hands. Remember: practice does not make perfect, it just makes permanent. Perfect practice makes perfect. Do not lay down faulty motor patterns with sloppy training.
- If the contact of the kettlebell on the forearm hurts, especially during cleans, snatches, presses and squats, consider using a sweatband to cushion it. You don't have to pass a 'trial by pain' period to allow you to use kettlebells. If it means that you can practice more frequently or engage in longer sessions, then I believe it is fine to use them.

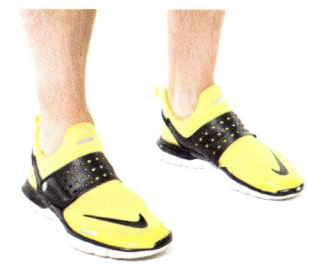

Figure 5.1 Nike Free training shoes

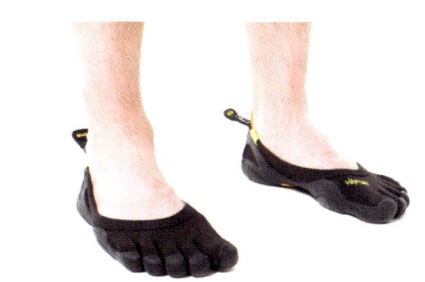

Figure 5.2 Vibram Five Fingers training shoes

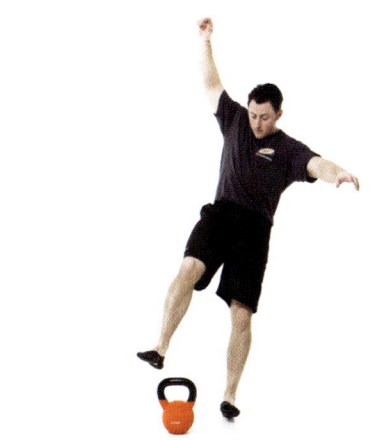

Figure 5.3 Place kettlebells in a safe place between sets in order to avoid the risk of injury

AFTER TRAINING

Safety considerations shouldn't come to an end just because your training session has.

- Cool down correctly by gradually lowering your heart rate and undertaking some static stretches.
- Over the sessions, look to build up training volume and intensity gradually.
- Take care of your hands by soaking them and/or smoothing/filing off calluses and moisturising the skin.

CONTRAINDICATIONS

There are numerous conditions for which kettlebell training may be inappropriate. Lower back pain, pregnancy, obesity, arthritis and hypertension are all examples of potential contraindications, but how they affect your training depends on the exercise being attempted and the individual circumstances. Even disc issues, such as bulging discs, don't always mean that you should never pick up a kettlebell. Please discuss any issues, injuries, medical conditions or diseases with your health practitioner (be it your doctor, specialist, physiotherapist and/or osteopath) to ensure that this type of training is suitable for you.

DIFFERENT GRIPS AND POSITIONS
6

There are many positions, stances and grips that should be mastered to ensure correct technique and efficiency when training with kettlebells. Performing the different grips and positions also provides sufficient variation and progression to stimulate improvements and changes (adaptations) within the body over a period of time.

SPINAL POSITION AND CORE ACTIVATION

The core muscles are the link between the upper and lower limbs. They stabilise the lumbar spine, the hips and the pelvis, as well as generate movement or decelerate the body or limbs. Fitness professionals and other related professionals, such as physiotherapists and sports massage therapists, use the term 'neutral spine' extensively. It describes the optimal positioning of the spine, particularly the lumbar spine, where the supporting structures (the ligaments and cartilage) are under minimal stress, and the central nervous system and muscles are expending minimal energy and tension to maintain this position. It is a position of optimal efficiency for both stabilisation and force production, and it limits undue stress on the tissues and structures that could cause injury. It is a position that should be practised during kettlebell training.

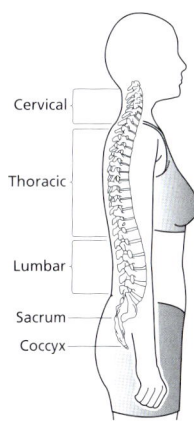

Figure 6.1 The neutral spine

MAINTAINING NEUTRAL SPINE POSITION

Simply speaking, the neutral spine position can be estimated by tilting the pelvis forwards (anterior tilt) and backwards (posterior tilt) until a mid-point is achieved. There should be a slight, but not excessive, curvature in the lower back. Lift the sternum up and try to elevate the head by 'standing tall'.

Common faults

Many people have poor body awareness and may only realise their level of proprioception when shown on video or in the mirror. Common faults include:

- allowing the pelvis to tilt forward, which can be due to tight hip flexors, weak or inactive hip extensors (glutes and hamstrings) and/or abdominals;
- rounding the upper back, which may be related to digestive dysfunction as it affects the body's ability to activate the core and stabilise the lower back and pelvis (when performing bent-over rows, deadlifts, squats or good mornings, some individuals round their back thinking that they are performing a hip hinge or pivot); and
- letting the sternum drop so that the upper back rounds over, which derives from individuals struggling to differentiate hip flexion (pivoting from the waist) and spinal flexion (rounding the back).

It is so important to ensure neutral spine position is achieved when training as a braced core in the correct position helps to transfer the force produced from the lower body or hips efficiently and effectively to the upper body and the load (the kettlebell). It can help to make you stronger during training and ensures you expel as little energy as possible lifting a weight (the definition of efficiency). It may also help to limit the risk of certain injuries. With the lower back in a flexed, loaded position, the risk of posterior migration of the intervertebral discs increases, which may cause a posterior bulging or even a prolapse of the discs, commonly referred to as a slipped disc. This bulging or prolapse can press on the nerves causing pain, functional restriction and even weakening the muscles that straighten the spine (spinal erectors) over a period of time.

To help prevent this it is important to learn, or to teach others, how to pivot from the hips and maintain an optimal back position as well as how to activate the core muscles correctly. Although previously the common recommendation was to hollow the abdomen (as if pulling the belly button towards the spine and making yourself thinner) and recruit the transversus abdominis (TVA), the standard recommendation with lifting loads, or when moderate to high levels of core activation are required, is to 'brace' the abdomen. This is akin to tensing the abdomen as if you were going to be punched in the stomach. The anterior and lateral core muscles should become taut when this bracing is initiated, and the posterior muscles of the lumbar back either side of the spinous processes should swell. The ribs and pelvis should remain still, and the 'connection' between the lower and upper body should be better. Although this technique is now taught, it is a natural instinct to brace when lifting, especially a heavy object, and each set of weightlifting should be initiated in this way. Do not try to tense your abdomen maximally as you don't need to do so with the weights that are used in kettlebell training, and anything more than required is simply a waste of energy. Don't push your stomach out and do not suck your stomach in as neither of these techniques help to support and protect your back effectively.

TYPE OF GRIPS

Figure 6.2 Rack with one hand

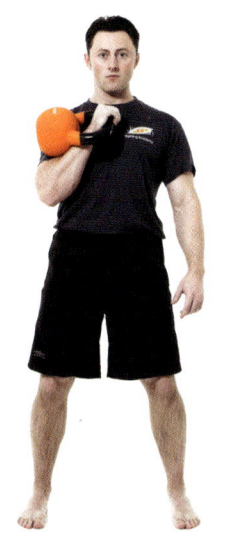

Figure 6.3 Bottoms up rack with one hand (or pistol grip)

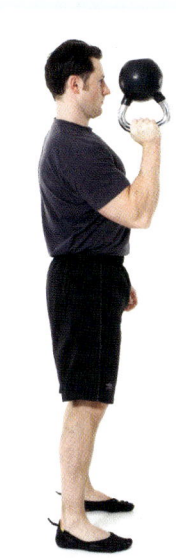

The rack is a position where the load is supported on or near the chest and shoulders. This is the starting and resting point for many exercises, including the clean, press, jerk and squat.

Execution
- Grip the handle, with the knuckle of the thumb on the pec (chest muscle).
- Keep the elbow close to the side near the hip.
- Rest the kettlebell on the forearm and the bicep.

This is a variation of the rack position. From this position a number of grip-emphasised drills can be undertaken, such as a squat, clean, press, curl or lunge.

Execution
- Hold the kettlebell in an upside-down position with the bell over the handle.
- Grip the handle tightly to stop the bell from falling or tipping to either side.
- *Note*: This is tough on the grip stabilisers of the hand, wrist and forearm.

Figure 6.4 Flipped rack with one hand (or waiter's hold)

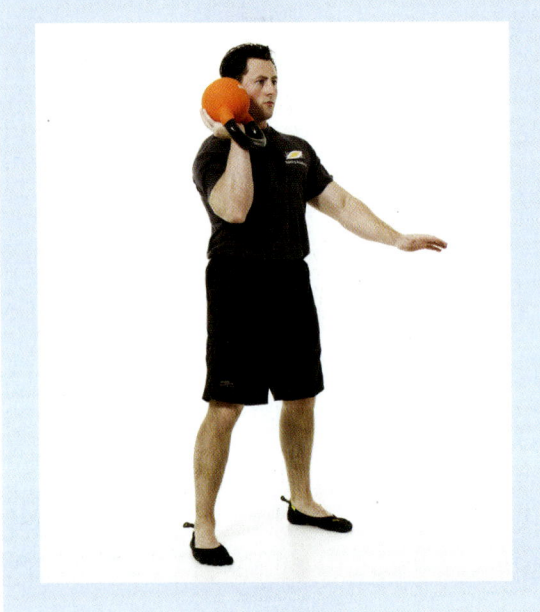

Figure 6.5 Bottoms up rack with two hands

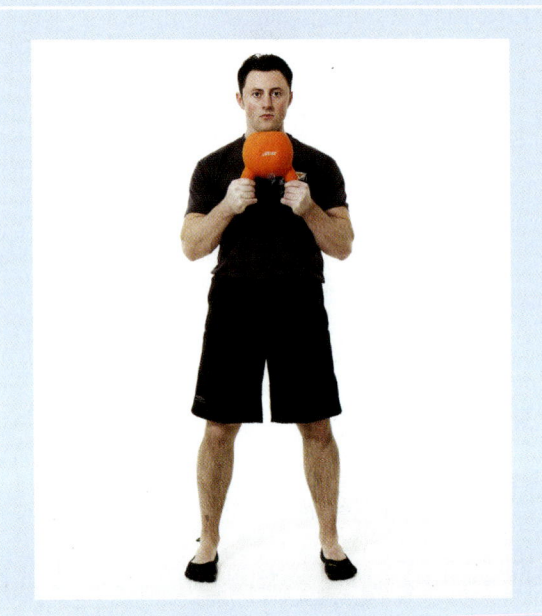

From this position a number of drills can be undertaken, such as a squat, clean, press, curl or step-up.

Execution
- Hold the kettlebell in an open-palm position by the bell section.
- Release the handle of the kettlebell and catch it near the shoulder with an open cupped palm.

This is a comfortable position for a front squat, two hand overhead press, squat-push press, lunge, get up anyhow, two hand curl or pistol squat.

Execution
- Hold the kettlebell by the horns, in an upside-down position, with the bell above the handle.
- Be sure to hold the bell close to the body.

Figure 6.6 Fingertip hold

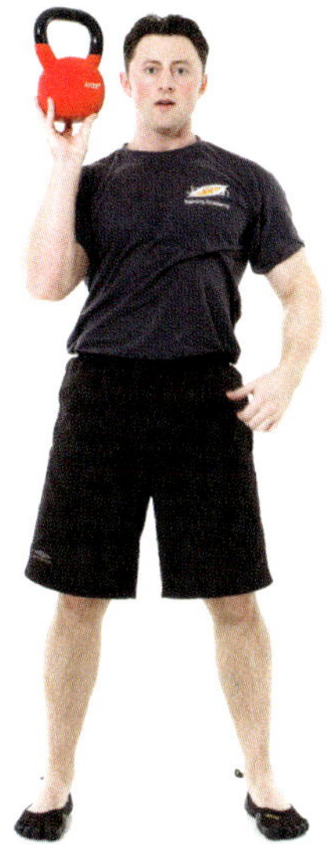

Figure 6.7 Farmer's hold

The fingertip hold requires strength in the fingers, just as doing a fingertip press-up. The drills using this grip are limited but you can squat, press or push press using this hold, however, the most common use is the overhead press.

Execution
- Hold one hand with the fingers and thumb facing upwards and place the kettlebell on top.
- Squeeze the edges of the bell of the kettlebell with the fingers and thumb to hold in place.

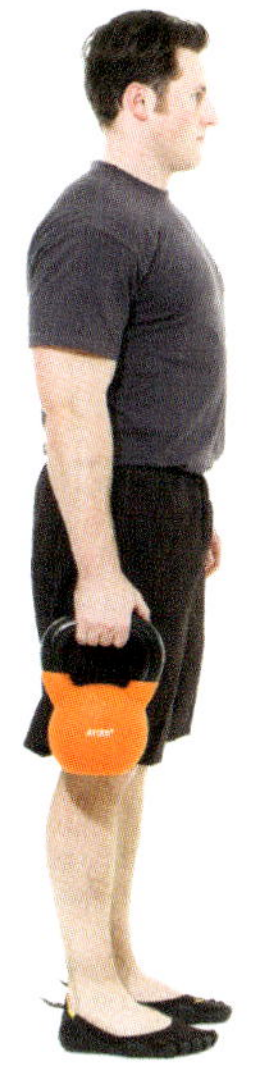

The farmer's hold is a simple position and is used for lunges, squats, suitcase deadlifts and, of course, the farmer's walk. Heavy and fat-grip kettlebells are good for use with this grip as it is tough on the forearm muscles when held for a longer period of time, which builds grip endurance.

Execution
- Hold the kettlebell by the handle at the side of the body by the hips. Thick handles will be more challenging for this grip.
- Hold two kettlebells in one hand to progress this drill or use a heavier bell.

Figure 6.8 Crush grip

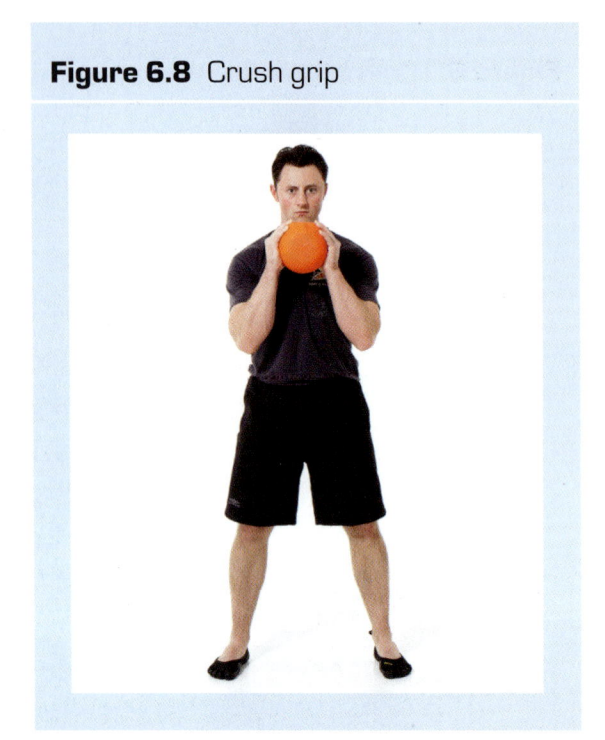

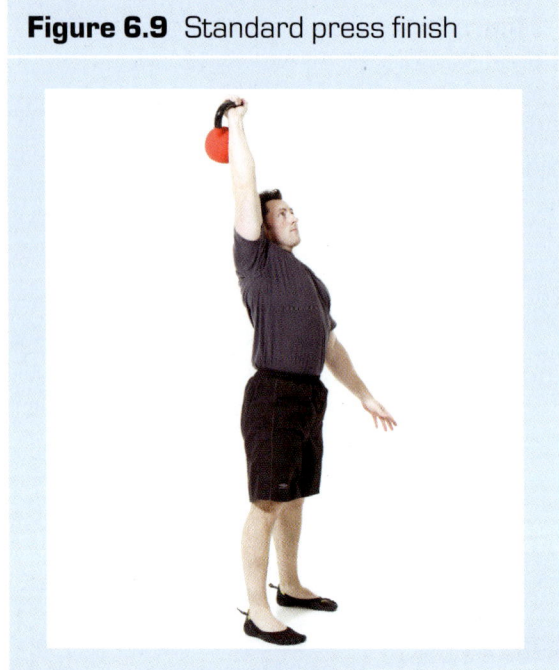

Figure 6.9 Standard press finish

Curls, squats, press, push press and lunges are all possible with this grip. Not the most common hold, but good as a variation to some of the exercises mentioned.

Execution
- Use both hands to grip the bell.
- Squeeze together to hold it in place.

This is a key position to master as it is required for many of the foundation drills, such as the snatch, the overhead press and the jerk. Many struggle with overhead positions because of limitations in mobility. An individual must be able to flatten the thoracic spine to accommodate the shoulder movement or they may find that the hand is too far forward or that the lower back over-arches (excessive lumber extension) to compensate.

Execution
- Hold the kettlebell with the handle across the palm and the bell on the forearms.
- Hold the handle directly above the shoulder, hips and ankle. The bell should actually sit slightly behind this line.
- This is the same for one or two-handed drills.

Figure 6.10 Dead position on floor between legs

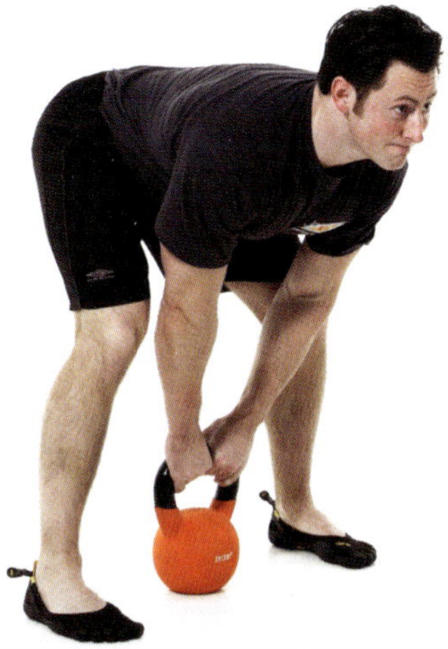

Figure 6.11 Dead position on floor in front of body

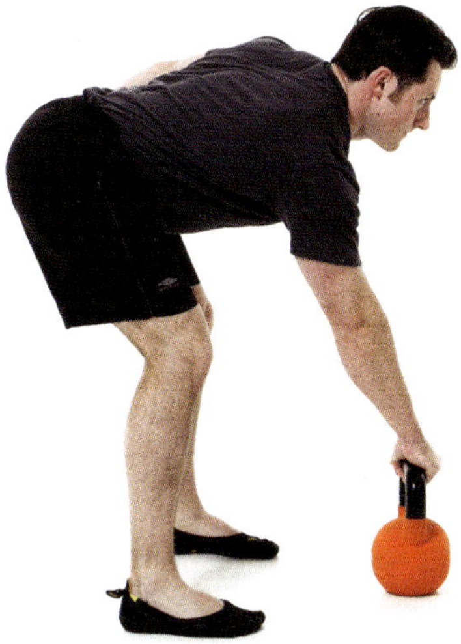

'Dead' simply means starting from a still position, without the dynamic, pre-loading eccentric phase. A dynamic eccentric phase, such as seen with a swing, stimulates the muscle spindles and allows for a utilisation of elastic energy to generate greater concentric force. Lifting from a dead start means that the mechanical sections only are used to generate the force to lift the weight. Holding for at least 4 seconds will eliminate all elastic energy.

Execution
- For most drills, position the bell in line with the heels to load the posterior chain muscles effectively.
- This position can be used for dead swings, dead cleans, dead snatches.

Many kettlebell enthusiasts like to initiate their swing, clean and snatch sets with the bell in front of their body. It is used as an alternative to starting with the bell on the hips and gently initiates the set with a 'mini-swing'. The negative aspect of this starting position is potential excessive loading on the structures of the lumbar spine may occur.

Execution
- Grip the bell with one or two hands.
- Forcefully pull it back between the legs to load the posterior chain muscles.
- Many start with the bell even further back than the position shown in figure 6.10.

Figure 6.12 Hang position

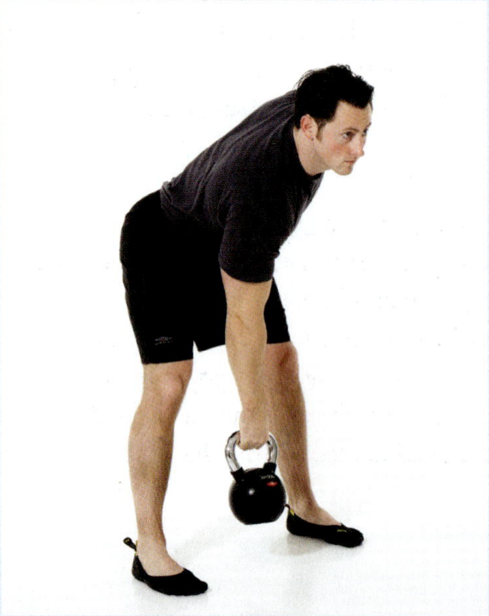

Figure 6.13 Two hand rack (or double rack)

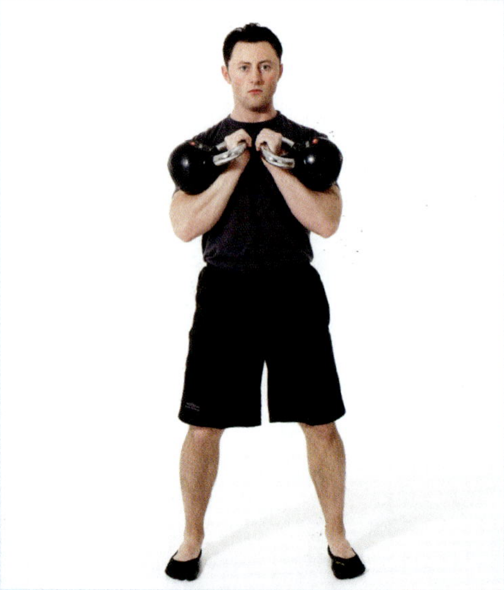

The hang position, as the name suggests, has the kettlebell hanging with the body in a semi-lifting position. This could be a low hang (see figure), a mid-hang with the bell between the knees, or a high hang position. Exercises could be dynamic where the bell is dropped to this position and then immediately lifted to the shoulder (rack) or overhead position, as during the snatch. A dead hang position is when the position is held for a few seconds to take the elastic energy out of the drill.

Execution
- Hold the kettlebell by the handle with the bell hanging downwards between the legs in an upright standing position.
- Squat down to the desired depth and execute the clean/snatch.

The two hand rack is a key position for competitive lifts such as the two kettlebell jerk and the two kettlebell long cycle jerk. The term long cycle means that between each repetition a swing clean is performed, for example, a long cycle squat means that the exercise is a clean and squat.

Execution
- The two hand rack is simply a double mirror version of the single hand rack.
- Hold the two kettlebells, one in each hand, in a double rack with the hands next to each other.

Figure 6.14 Two hand rack Girevoy style

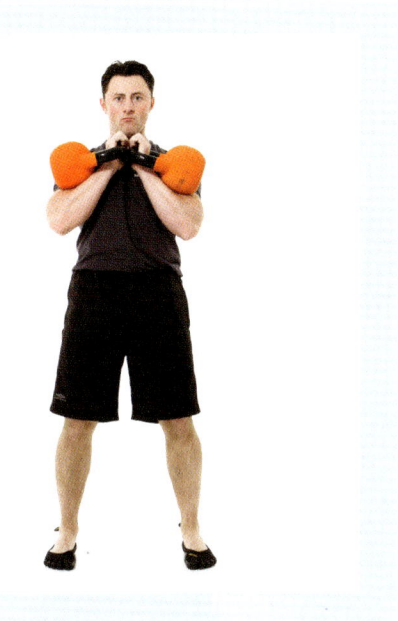

The Girevoy style (GS) version of the double rack involves more rounding of the upper back so that the elbows 'rest' on the hips and the fingers are tucked behind the handle. The reason for this is to avoid any potential finger crushing that could occur if the bell handles bang together.

Execution
- Employ more of a rounded back.
- Rest your elbows on your hips and tuck your fingers behind the handle.
- As in the overhead press finish position, the fingers do not need to grip the handle of the bell in the rack as the handle is held across the palm and in place by the thumb.

2

PART **TWO**

THE EXERCISES

KETTLEBELL WARM-UP

An effective warm-up is essential to any training programme, but especially when training with kettlebells. Kettlebell lifting is demanding on the entire body and it is critical that it has been well prepared for the dynamic nature of many of these exercises. For individuals to be able to undertake the session effectively and without exposing the body structures to an increased risk of injury, a comprehensive warm-up up to 10 minutes or more must be completed.

Although the term 'warm-up' is used, increasing the body's temperature is just one outcome of an effective and comprehensive warm-up. One could sit in a sauna for 10 minutes to increase the body temperature, but that does not sufficiently prepare the body for a session of swings, snatches and cleans. The warm-up should:

- increase the body temperature;
- mobilise all the joints to be used in the session; and
- prepare the neuromuscular system for the session intensity.

This means that lower intensity mobilisation drills, as well as dynamic drills that mimic the planned exercises, should be incorporated within the warm-up, preferably in the following order for maximum effectiveness:

1. Low-intensity mobilisation drills
2. Loaded mobilisation drills
3. Dynamic mobilisation drills

Limited mobility

There are certain trends that personal trainers and physiotherapists across the Western world see regularly in their clients and patients: limited mobility in the foot or ankle, hips and in the thoracic spine. Limited mobility in any of these areas impairs the optimal range of motion when squatting. Limited mobility in the hips affects the lifting pattern of the clean, snatch and swing, while restrictions in the thoracic spine may impede an effective overhead pressing pattern. Since many of the foundation kettlebell drills are built around the lift pattern, focus on the hips in the warm-up to ensure optimal mobility and function. However, the other areas should not be ignored.

1. LOW-INTENSITY MOBILISATION DRILLS

Perform 10–15 repetitions of each mobilisation drill. Do not hold the end range, as is common for static stretches, but simply move through the range as instructed in a slow and controlled manner.

Figure 7.1 Neck mobility

(a) (b)

Figure 7.2 Angry cat

(a)

(b)

Execution
- Rotate the chin slowly from one side to the other, briefly pausing for half a second at the end range.
- Then drop the ear to the shoulder, alternating sides. Avoid shrugging the shoulders.
- Finish by dropping the chin to the chest, trying to 'lengthen the spine' as you do this.

This drill is to mobilise the structures of the spine, especially good if you have been seated or immobile (sleeping) for a long period prior to the session.

Execution
- On all fours, allow the lower back to sag, tilting the hips forwards.
- Without holding, flex the spine to round the back, tilting the hips backwards.
- Keep the head in line with the spine and move through this extension-flexion pattern in a slow and controlled fashion.

Figure 7.3 Fire hydrant

(a)

(b)

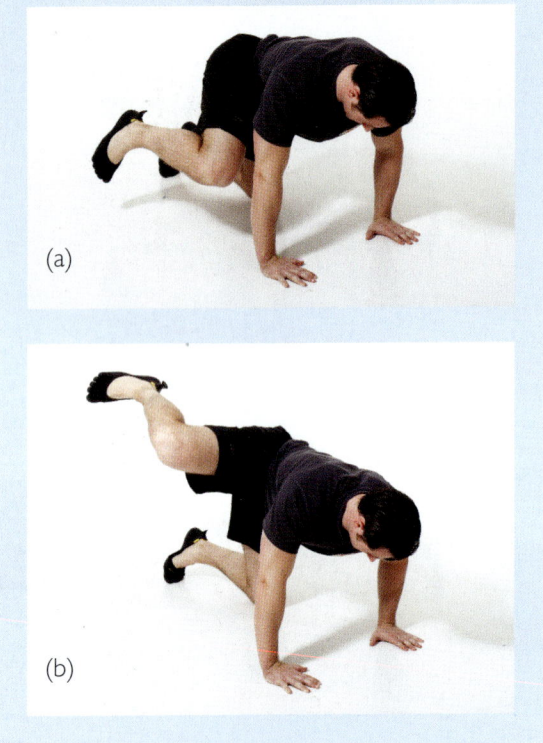

Figure 7.4 Spiderman stretch

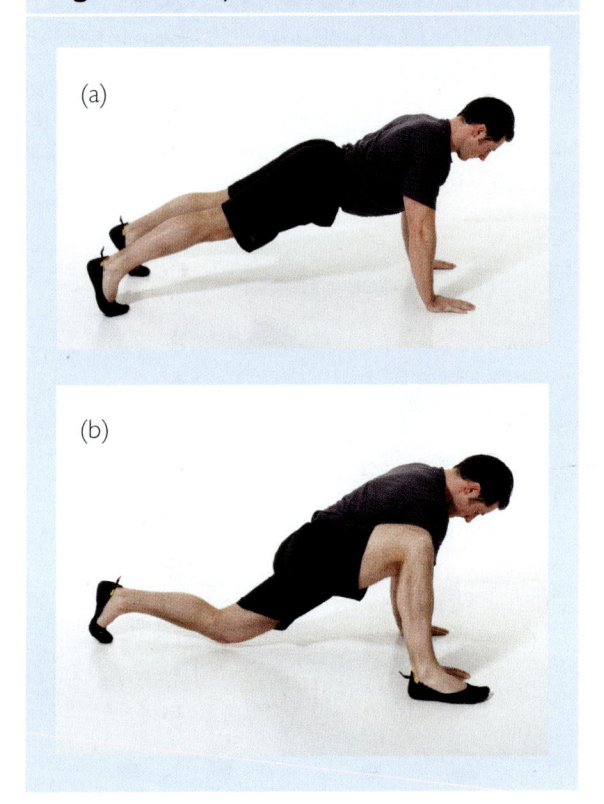

(a)

(b)

Execution
- Start on all fours in the angry cat position (see figure 7.2, page 35).
- Lift one knee off the ground without shifting your weight and bring the knee up and out to the side. Hold briefly then repeat on the same side before switching.
- Then, in the same position, repeat the drill but using a circular motion with the knee. This is good for getting some mobility at the commonly tight hip joint.

This drill is fantastic for opening the tight hip flexors, which can limit the swing, clean and snatch exercises.

Execution
- Adopt the plank position.
- Then, lift one foot upwards and place to the outside of the ipsilateral (same side) hand and hold.
- Gently drop the knee towards the floor, and lift the hands off the ground and above the head leaning back (not shown).
- Gently rock back and forth, then return to the start position and repeat on the other side.

Figure 7.5 Prayer upward-facing dog

(a)

(b)

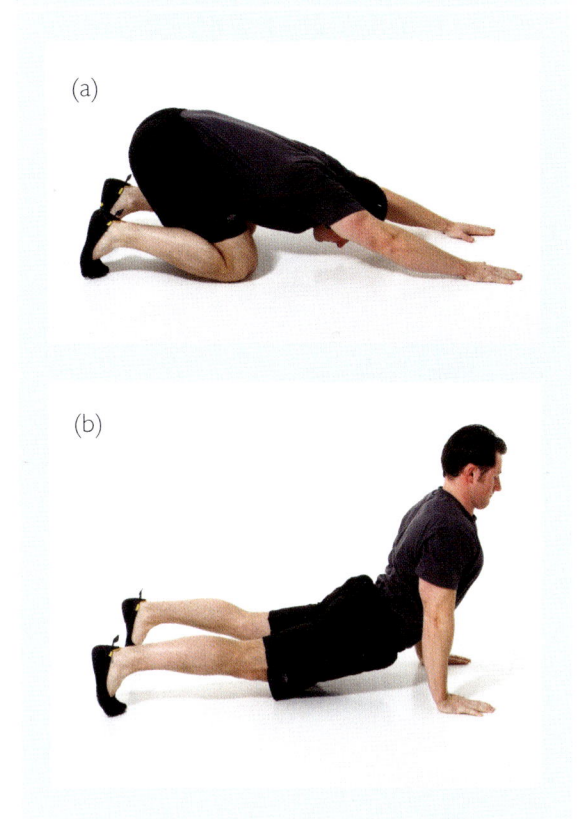

Figure 7.6 Supine bridge

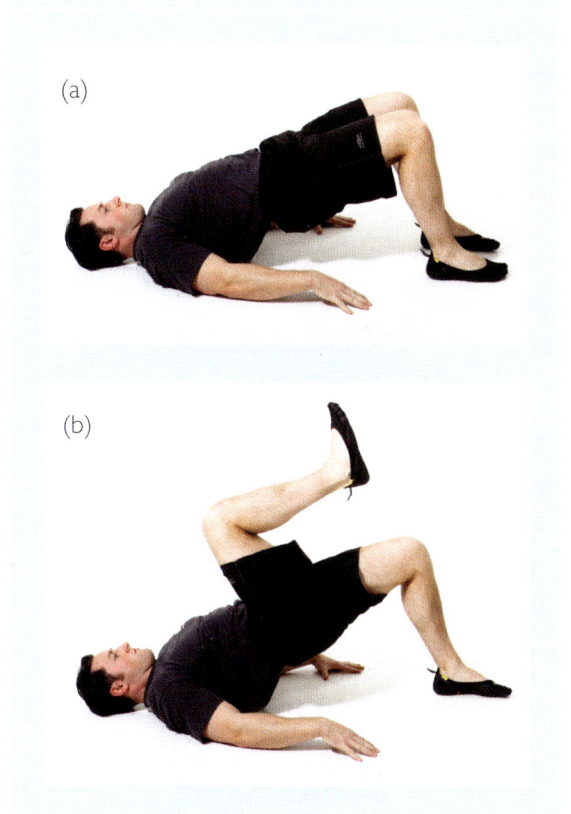

(a)

(b)

Execution
- On all fours, sit back onto the heels and push upwards with the arms.
- Then, push the hips forwards, until the shoulders are over the hands, extending through the arms and keeping the hips low to the ground.
- Move smoothly and slowly through these two positions repeatedly.

Execution
- Lie in a supine position on the floor (facing the ceiling), with the knees bent and the feet close to the hips.
- Focus on the glutes and contract to lift the hips off the floor until full extension is reached and the knees, hips and shoulders are in a straight line.
- Lower the hips to the ground, but do not allow touching or relaxing. Repeat this action. This can also be undertaken in a single leg format (see figure 7.6b) with the other knee pulled towards the chest.

Figure 7.7 Inchworm

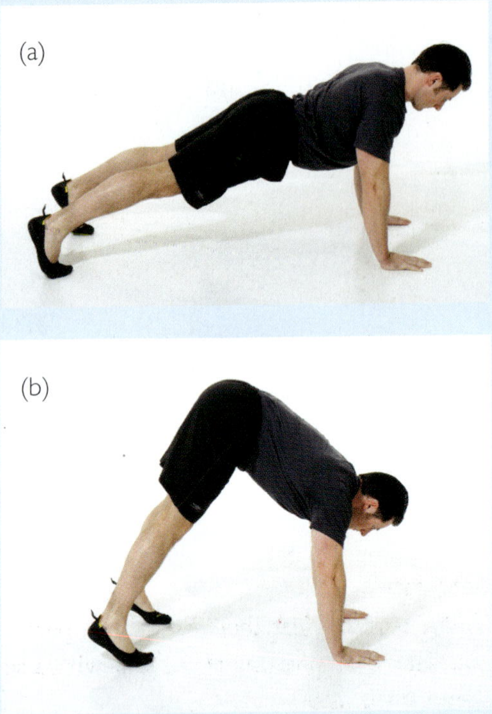

(a)

(b)

Execution
- Start in the plank position then, keeping the core engaged and the legs straight, 'walk' the feet forwards towards the hands until tension is felt in the hamstrings.
- From this position then walk the hands forwards back to a plank position.
- Repeat for a set distance or 10–15 repetitions.

Figure 7.8 Knee to chest

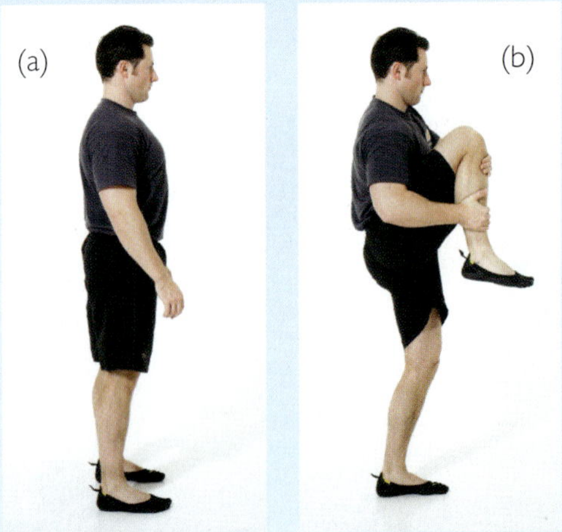

(a)   (b)

Execution
- Stand on one leg then lift the other leg and bring the knee towards the chest.
- Hold the knee briefly with the arms then return to the start position and repeat on the opposite side.
- Try to keep the chest up throughout to prevent the back from rounding over.

Figure 7.9 Hip rotation

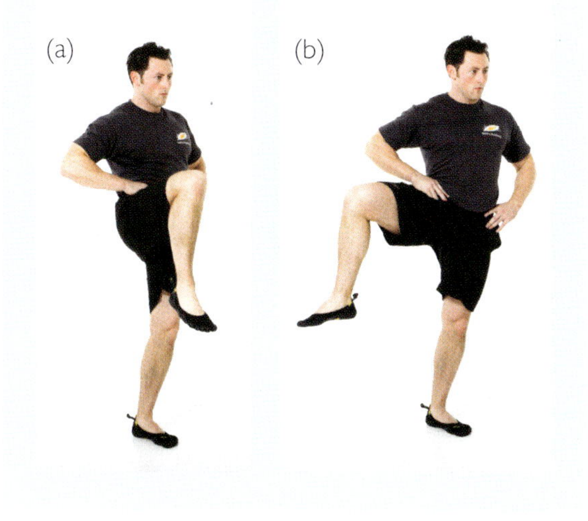

(a) (b)

Figure 7.10 Romanian deadlift (or hip hinge/waiter's bow)

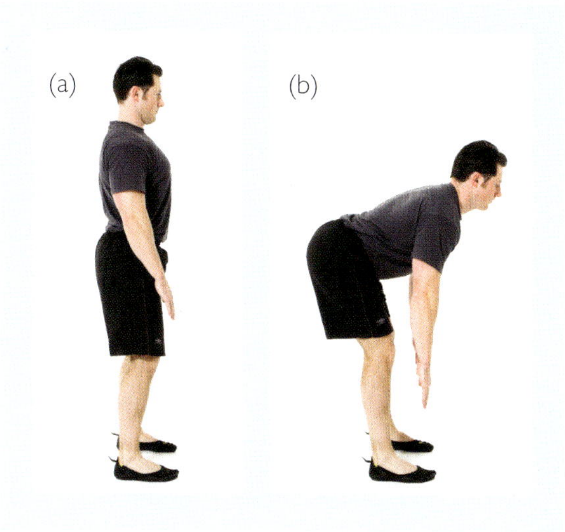

(a) (b)

Execution
- Stand on one leg then lift one knee upwards then outwards to mobilise the hip joint.
- Repeat for 10–15 repetitions, then change direction bringing the knee outwards and then in and downwards.
- Repeat on both sides.

Execution
- Stand with the feet about hip width apart.
- Bow forward, pivoting at the hips with a slight bend at the knee.
- Push the hips back and tip the pelvis forward to maintain a neutral spine and optimal back alignment. Bend forwards enough until tension is felt in the hamstrings. Hands should be about mid-upper shin height.
- Push the hips forward and return to the start position.

Figure 7.11 Single leg Romanian deadlift (SLRDL)

(a)

(b)

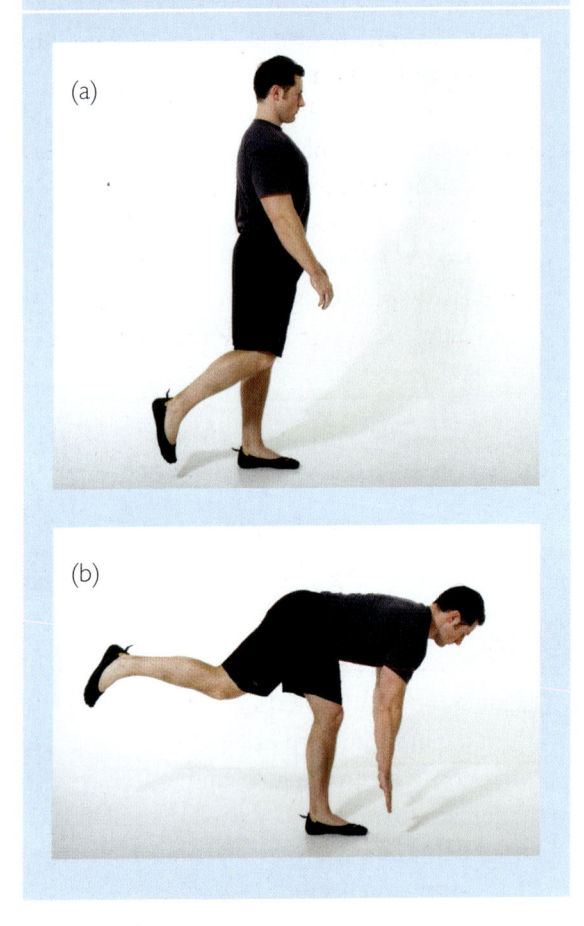

Figure 7.12 Quad stretch SLRDL

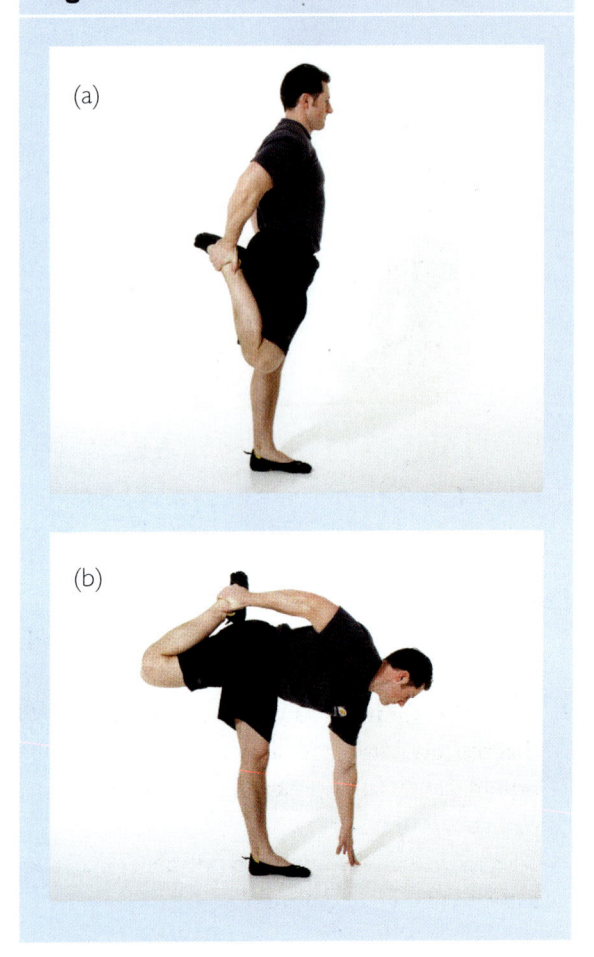

(a)

(b)

Execution
- Stand on one leg then pivot forwards from the hips, extending the rear leg behind and reaching down to touch the front foot.
- Keep the chest up and the front leg stiff.
- Extend the rear leg back to help tilt the pelvis forward and apply the stretch to the hamstrings and to maintain balance.
- Keep the hands off the floor and away from the leg and use the hip stabilisers to maintain balance.

Execution
- Stand on one leg then bring the heel to the glute and hold with the ipsilateral (same side) hand.
- Pivot forwards from the hips, extending the rear leg behind and reaching down to touch the front foot, with the same side hand.
- Keep the chest up throughout.

Figure 7.13 Reverse crossover lunge

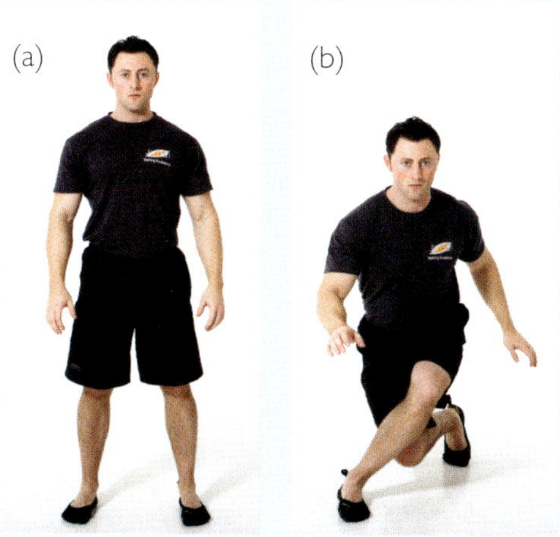

(a)   (b)

Execution
- Stand with feet about hip to shoulder width apart.
- With the right leg, step back and behind so that the foot hits diagonally at a southwest angle.
- Squat down on the left leg and perform a curtsy-type motion.
- Keep hips facing forward to optimally load and activate the hip abductors.

SCIATIC NERVE MOBILISATION

Many of the key kettlebell drills (swings, snatches, cleans) rely on a correct lift-pattern and optimal function of the muscles involved in this action. The sciatic nerve is a controlling nerve for many of the muscles involved in producing force for a lift, and if it is not functioning optimally, it may cause tension in the low back, Piriformis tightness and hamstring hypertonicity. This nerve mobilisation technique was shown to me by physiotherapist and biomechanics expert Martin Haines, and has proved to be very effective for most people in diminishing the issues associated with the sciatic nerve and kettlebell training, such as low back muscular tension, hamstrings spasms and hip flexion range of motion.

Note: For some individuals with an irritated sciatic nerve, this mobilisation technique may aggravate symptoms, in which case cease the drill. However, most coaches that use this technique do find it to be very effective for the majority of clients that present with the issues mentioned above or that have a positive test on the straight leg raise test (sciatic nerve).

Figure 7.14 Sciatic nerve mobilisation

(a)

(b)

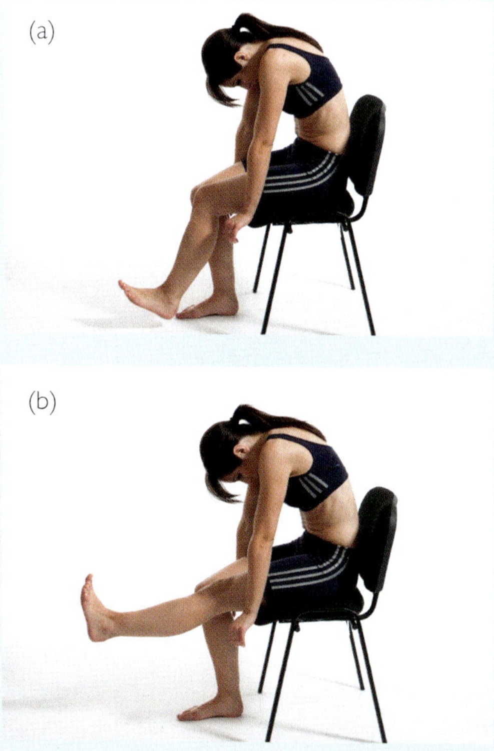

Execution
- Sit on the end of a wall, bench or couch. A chair can be used (as shown) but it is better if both legs are hanging down and not touching the floor.
- Place the chin on the chest and slump the upper body over as far as possible.
- On the left leg, pull the toes to the shin (dorsiflexion) and then holding that position at the ankle, perform a leg extension and straighten the leg at the knee. Stop at the point of tension.
- Then, bend the knee slightly, enough to take the tension off, and straighten again.
- Perform 10–15 repetitions then change legs.
- Repeat 3-4 times on each leg, four times a day (including before and after any exercise session).

2. LOADED MOBILISATION DRILLS

All exercises should be performed for a minimum of 10 reps on each side. Warming up should always be an integral part of any kettlebell training session and these mobilising exercises should raise the heart rate, mobilise the joints and raise the temperature. Spend about 10 minutes undertaking the following drills as well as bodyweight or lightweight versions of the kettlebell exercises to be trained within the session.

Perform these mobilisation drills with a kettlebell of an appropriate weight for each position. Do not assume that all drills should be completed with the same weight of kettlebell that you use in your exercise session, usually it is best to use the next weight down. If a 16kg kettlebell is going to be used for the session, then warm up with a 12kg or 8kg bell.

Figure 7.15 Kettlebell around the body pass

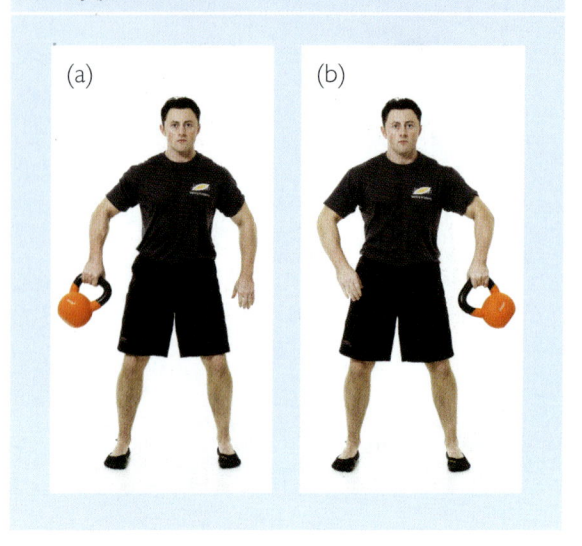

(a) (b)

Execution
- Holding the kettlebell by the handle, swing the bell around the body at waist height, keeping the shoulders and hips as still as possible.
- Practice swapping the hands in front and behind the body as smoothly and effortlessly as possible.
- Swing for 10–15 repetitions in both directions.
- Practise with the eyes closed for an additional challenge.

Figure 7.16 Kettlebell halos

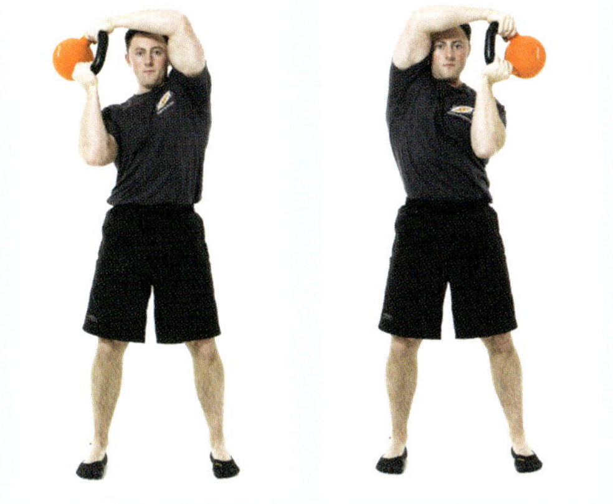

(a) (b)

Figure 7.17 Kettlebell good morning

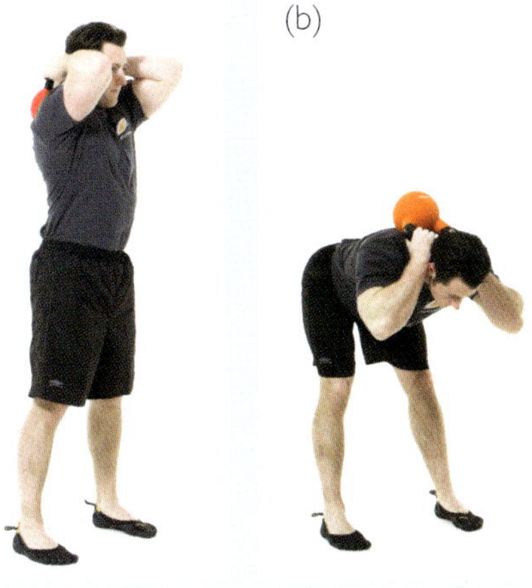

(a) (b)

Execution
- Hold the kettlebell in a two hand bottoms-up position in front of the face.
- Keeping the kettlebell close to the head, roll the elbow across and over the head so that the kettlebell goes behind and then round the other side.
- Repeat in both directions, trying to maintain a solid position with the hips and upper torso.

Execution
- Hold either one kettlebell by the handle with both hands, or two kettlebells, one in each hand. Hold so that the kettlebell rests on the upper back and not the neck.
- Push the hips back, keeping the knees stiff but not locked, and the chest high.
- Bend forward as far as possible from the waist, keeping the spine neutral and avoiding rounding over.
- Return to the start position using the glutes to straighten the body and repeat.

Figure 7.18 Kettlebell figure-of-eight between legs

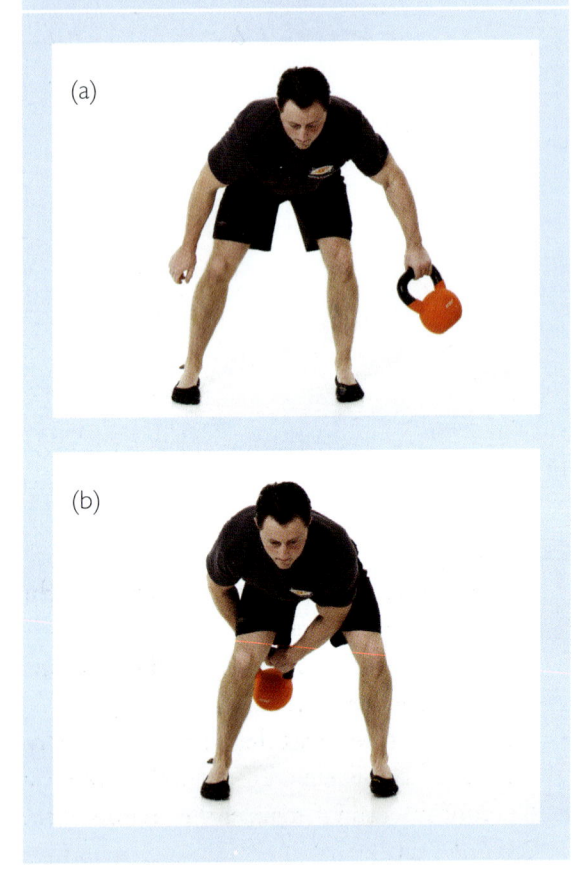

(a)

(b)

Figure 7.19 Kettlebell arm bar

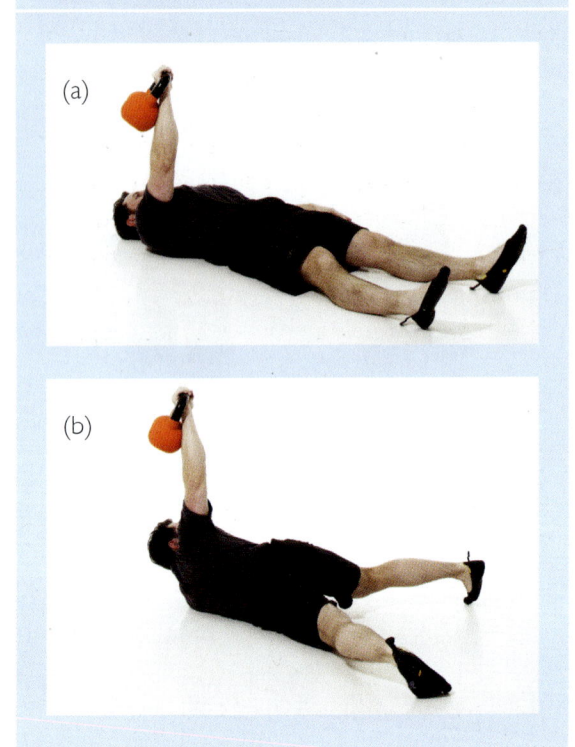

(a)

(b)

This is a good warm-up drill for many of the supine exercises, such as the Turkish get-up, as it mobilises the shoulder under load.

Execution
- Stand with the legs shoulder width apart or slightly wider.
- Swing the kettlebell diagonally between the legs, swap hands and bring the kettlebell around the leg.
- Swing diagonally between the legs and around and repeat. Continue this figure-of-eight pattern for 10 reps in each direction.

Execution
- Start in a supine position with the kettlebell held in one hand above the body with the arm extended.
- Slowly lift the leg on the same side up and over to touch the floor on the other side and roll the body as this is done.
- Keep the arm vertical throughout and only go as far as the shoulder mobility allows.

3. DYNAMIC MOBILISATION DRILLS

It is recommended that you include some dynamic stretches within the warm-up to help increase the heart rate and temperature, and to mobilise the joints at a quicker velocity. Static stretches have not been shown to help reduce injuries before a training session, and they may in fact reduce the strength and power of the muscles by initiating an inhibiting and relaxing effect. This is fine for post-exercise stretching, but it is not helpful for pre-exercise mobilisation.

Figure 7.20 Lunge and overhead reach

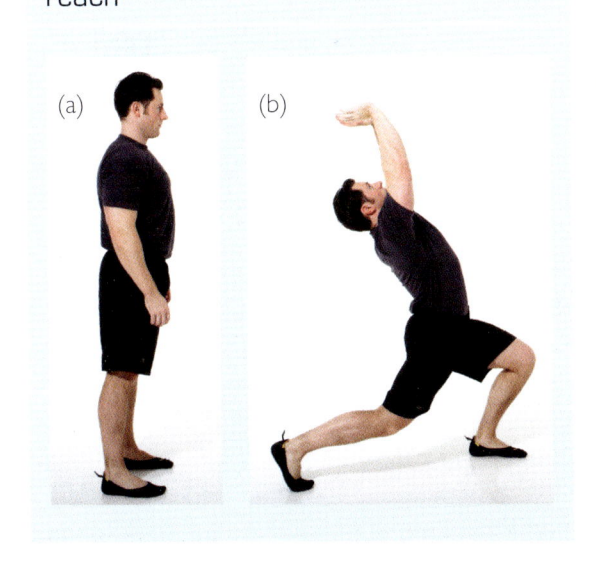

Figure 7.21 Lunge and rotation

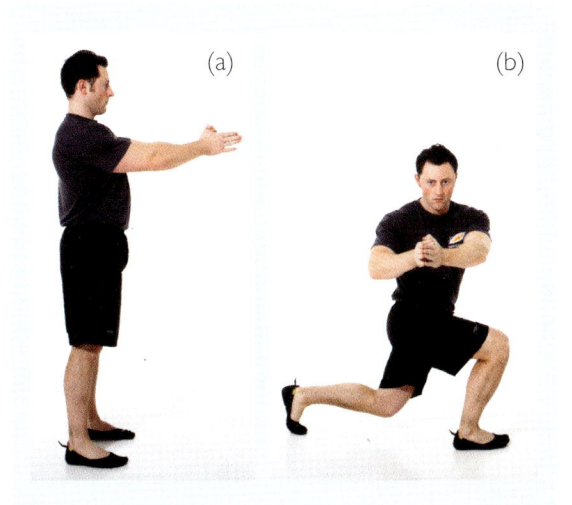

Execution
- Stand with feet about hip width apart and the arms extended in front.
- Take a longer than normal step forward and drop into a lunge position.
- At the same time, twist the torso and rotate the arms over the bent leg. This mobilises the rear leg hip flexors and stimulates the rotators of the core (obliques).
- Push back to the start position and repeat on both sides.

Execution
- Stand with feet about hip width apart.
- Take a longer than normal step forward and drop into a lunge position.
- At the same time, reach overhead and back with the arms to mobilise the rear leg hip flexors and to stimulate the anterior core (rectus abdominis).
- Push back to the start position and repeat on both sides.

Figure 7.22 Bodyweight squat

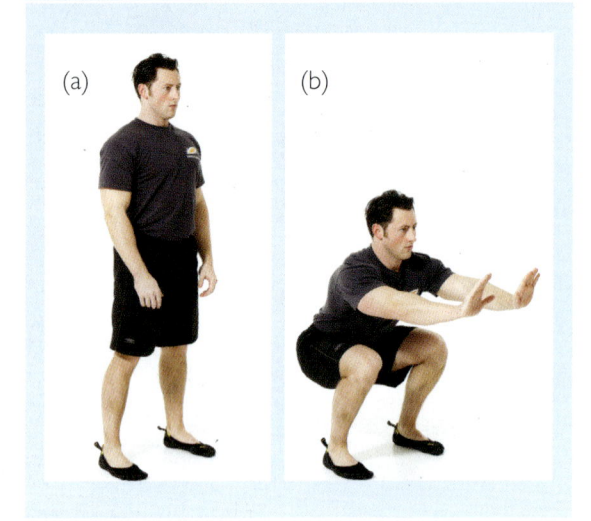

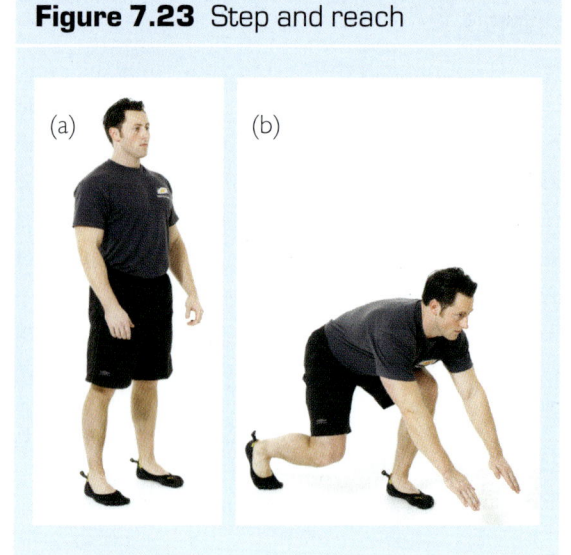

Figure 7.23 Step and reach

Execution
- Stand with feet about hip to shoulder width apart, pointing forward or slightly rotated out.
- Bend from the knees and hips and squat down as low as possible, keeping the shins and upper torso parallel.
- Push back up to the start position and repeat.
- Keep the feet flat on the ground and the chest up throughout.

Execution
- Stand with feet about hip width apart, arms by the sides. Take a normal step forward (shorter than a lunge) and reach forwards and downwards with the arms, as if picking something up.
- Keep the front shin vertical (imperative), as if reaching over a small fence, to load the hamstrings and glutes effectively.
- The chest should be up and the spine neutral throughout the drill.
- Push back up to the start and repeat.

Figure 7.24 Sagittal leg swings

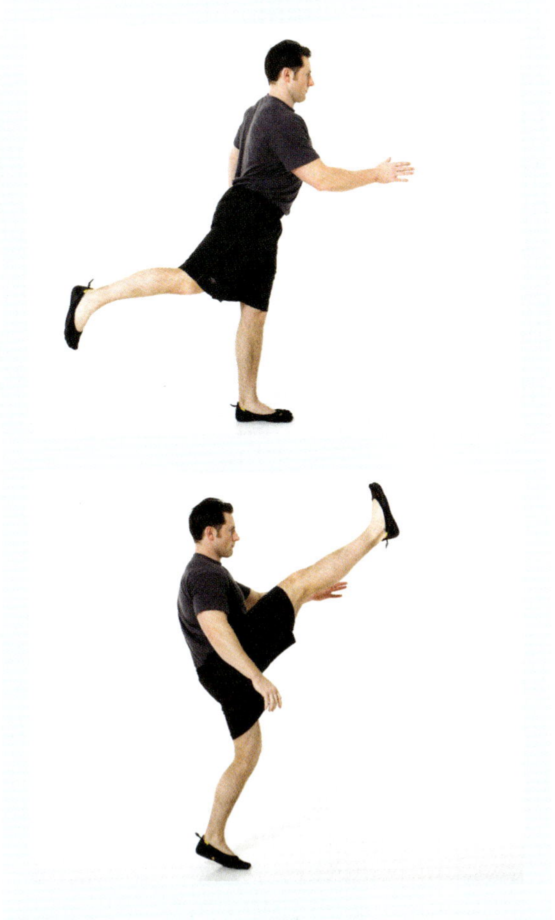

Figure 7.25 Frontal leg swings

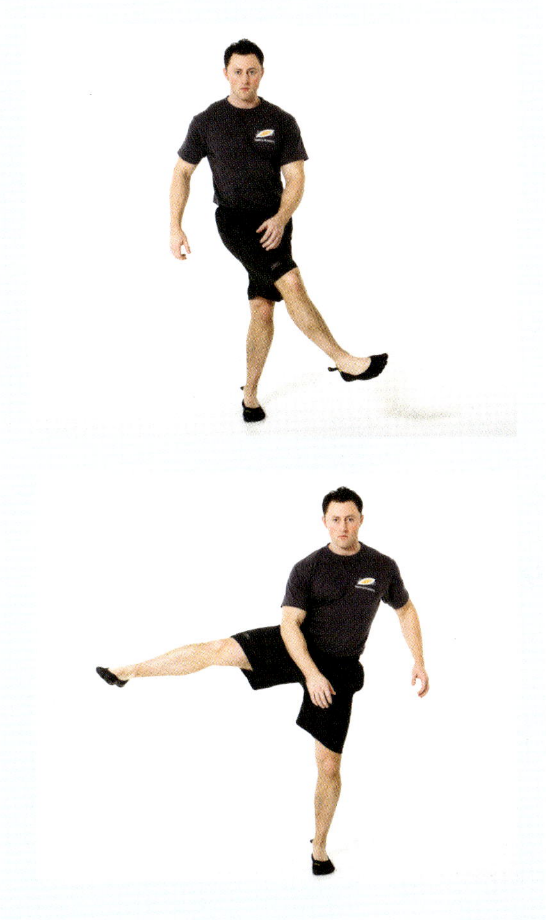

Execution
- Stand on one leg then swing the other leg forward, touching the knee/shin/foot with the opposite hand.
- Swing the leg back and, if you can without losing balance, reach upwards and backwards with the opposite arm.
- Increase the range of movement (ROM) slightly with each repetition and repeat on the other side.

Execution
- Stand on one leg.
- Then, swing the other leg across the body.
- Swing the leg back across and outwards, maintaining the balance with the arms.
- Increase the ROM slightly with each repetition and repeat on the other side.

PREPARATION EXERCISES

8

These exercises allow the kettlebell user to develop the necessary mobility, technique and basic strength to successfully complete the kettlebell drills described later in this book.

THE BODYWEIGHT SQUAT

The squat is a fundamental human movement pattern and the parallel stance squat is a prerequisite for all of the other squat pattern movements, which include the split stance squat, lunge, single leg squat, step-up, jump and hop. There is much debate about the correct method of squatting, such as whether the knees should move forward of the toes or stay behind, how far apart the feet should be and what is the correct depth at which to perform a squat.

DEPTH

It has been a common misconception for a number of years that the ideal depth for squatting is 90 degrees or thighs parallel to the floor. These recommendations came about after research proposed that full depth squats, where the hamstrings touch the calves, potentially increased knee instability and caused knee health issues later in life (Klein, 1962). Further investigations and research reviews undertaken by the National Strength and Conditioning Association (NSCA) in the early 1990s (Chandler & Stone, 1991) have since shown these conclusions to be unfounded. There is inherently no reason why an individual cannot undertake full depth squats, including loaded (holding a kettlebell), unless that individual experiences pain or has pre-existing conditions that may inhibit them or that could be worsened with this exercise. If the individual cannot maintain a neutral spine position or a flat back throughout the range without rounding over, the range of motion should be limited.

KNEES

During a squat the load or stress should be equally distributed throughout the joints that perform that movement pattern. If one joint has less stress placed upon it, then the other joints have to undergo more stress to compensate. For example, if the knees are deliberately kept back and knee flexion is restricted, then the body flexes more from the hips and the upper torso leans further forward to maintain balance over the base of support. This causes less stress to be placed upon the knee, but creates more load and stress on the spine and the structures and tissue that support it.

To optimally distribute the load between the knees, hips and spine, the torso and shins should be roughly parallel with each other throughout the movement. Avoid deliberately keeping the knees back and the question of whether they should move beyond the toes or not will depend on the individual's biomechanics, such as the length of their tibia and the size of their feet.

FOOT POSITION

The squat pattern should be performed with an athletic stance, such as that adopted for a vertical jump. The feet can be rotated up to approximately 30 degrees, but anything more than that is usually indicative of tight hip rotators, either on one foot or both feet, depending on what is seen.

Many individuals with very tight feet or ankles naturally and subconsciously adopt a wider stance to perform squats to compensate for these restrictions. With a wider stance, less dorsiflexion is required and the flexibility issues are not so apparent. Try to keep the stance athletic, even if it means limiting the range of motion in the short term, and look to address the flexibility issues with stretching, myofascial release with sports massage or other techniques such as rolfing or active release techniques, and self-myofascial release using a foam roller or similar implement.

TECHNIQUE

Before loading the body with weights, such as a kettlebell, it is important that the appropriate technique and mobility for this movement pattern are acquired. The squat works predominantly the quadriceps, hamstrings, glutes and stabilisers of the foot, ankle, knee and hip. When performing this exercise, the knee flexes, the hips flex and the ankle dorsiflexes as the body 'folds' at these joints under the weight of gravity. These muscles then contract and shorten to create the triple extension of the concentric phase of the squat pattern (extension at the hip, extension at the knee and plantarflexion at the ankle).

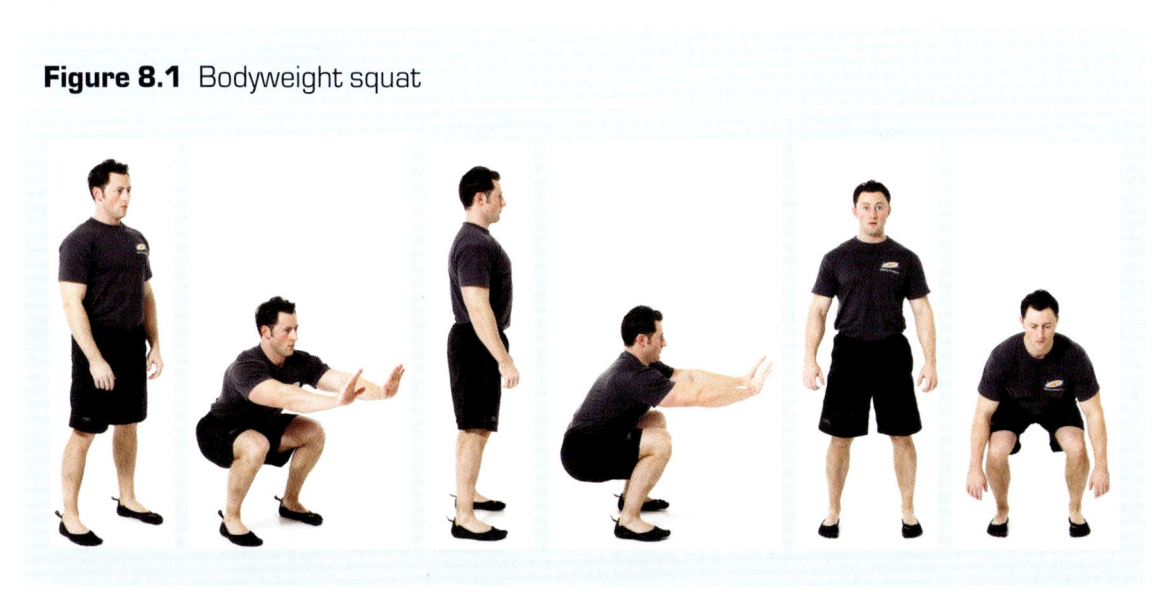

Figure 8.1 Bodyweight squat

Execution
- Stand with feet hip to shoulder width apart and pointing forwards or rotated out to a maximum of 30 degrees.
- Push the knees forward and bend forward from the waist to lower the hips towards the heels.
- Squat down as low as possible, keeping the chest up, the spine neutral or flat and the feet flat on the ground.
- Push the hips forward to straighten the knees and hips and drive through the feet to press the body back up to the start position.

THE BARBELL OVERHEAD SQUAT

The progression from the bodyweight squat is the weighted overhead squat. The weight does not have to be a 20kg Olympic bar (as shown in figure 8.2), but could be a fit bar or even an adjustable studio barbell. The additional challenge of holding a bar above the head and keeping the bar over the feet requires optimal mobility in the hips and shoulders and helps to show if the upper torso is leaning too far forward. The hands should be positioned shoulder width apart on the bar or slightly further along. Squat down as low as possible to evaluate how the body undertakes this task. Look for the following:

- If the heels lift up, this indicates restrictions in the foot or ankle and limited dorsiflexion.
- Knees caving in indicates poor knee or hip stability.
- Being unable to achieve a full range of motion (full squat) indicates limitations in the foot, ankle or hip.
- The bar coming forward of the toes indicates either limited thoracic mobility, tight shoulders (particularly the muscles that medially rotate the shoulder) or restrictions in the foot, ankle or hip, causing issues further up the kinetic chain.

Common advice is that individuals should be able to successfully complete this test or exercise before undertaking certain drills, such as overhead pressing. If thoracic mobility is limited, then that individual will struggle to get the arms straight up above the head without having to compensate somewhere else, such as anteriorly tilting the pelvis forward and overarching the lumbar spine (lower back).

Figure 8.2 Barbell overhead squat

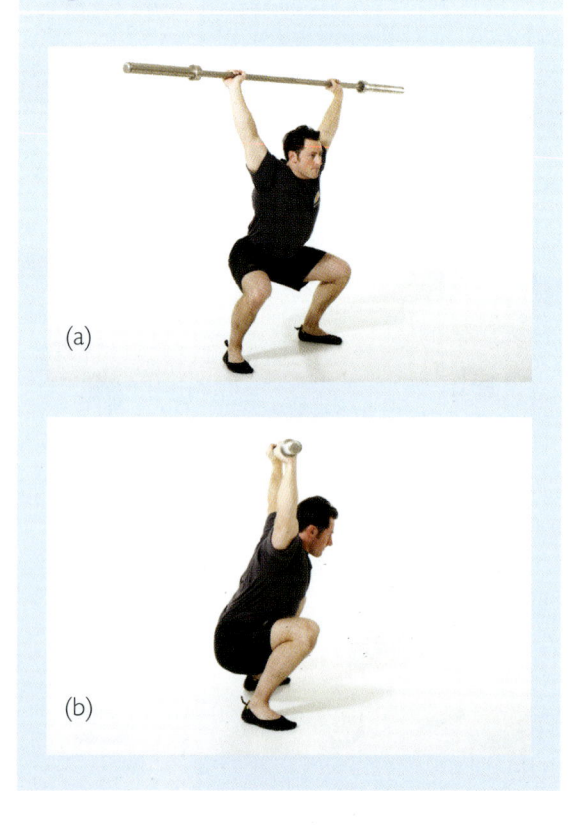

(a)

(b)

THE BARBELL ROMANIAN DEADLIFT (RDL)

The loaded Romanian deadlift should be preceded with the bodyweight Romanian deadlift, also known as the hip hinge or waiter's bow. An individual should be able to 'hinge' at the hips and have what some authors refer to as hip-back disassociation. This means that they can flex or bend at the hips, whilst not flexing or bending at the spine and maintaining a normal lumbar curvature (neutral spine) or flat back. If the individual rounds the back, then this has the potential to excessively load the structures of the spine and could cause injury.

Figure 8.3 Barbell RDL

(a) (b)

(c)

Once the individual can demonstrate this technique unloaded, they can progress to performing this hip hinge with a weight, such as a barbell.

Execution
- Hold the bar with hands slightly wider than hip width apart and feet about hip width apart.
- Push the hips back and lean forward, maintaining an optimal back position and avoiding rounding over.
- Lower the bar to approximately mid-shin height or as far as possible with good technique, then squeeze the glutes and pull the hips forward to lift the bar back to the start position.

THE BODYWEIGHT SIDE PLANK

The side plank is a common exercise seen in many gyms, fitness centres and health clubs. It works the lateral core muscles (the internal and external obliques) and the lateral hip muscles to improve frontal plane stability and endurance. Healthy individuals should be able to hold the lateral or side plank on the elbow for about 80–90 seconds at least on each side with a maximum of 5 per cent difference between sides (McGill, 2002). This exercise helps to provide the stability required when lifting a weight with one hand (suitcase-style deadlift or a farmer's walk) and pressing a weight overhead with one hand (kettlebell one hand overhead press). This non-functional exercise can therefore have a positive functional carryover during pressing, lifting and moving or carrying loads using one side.

This exercise can be performed on the elbow or with the arm straight (see both methods in figure 8.4). The straight-arm variation requires more shoulder stability; so many individuals prefer the elbow or forearm version to focus on the lateral core and not to be inhibited by shoulder stability limitations.

Figure 8.4 Bodyweight side plank

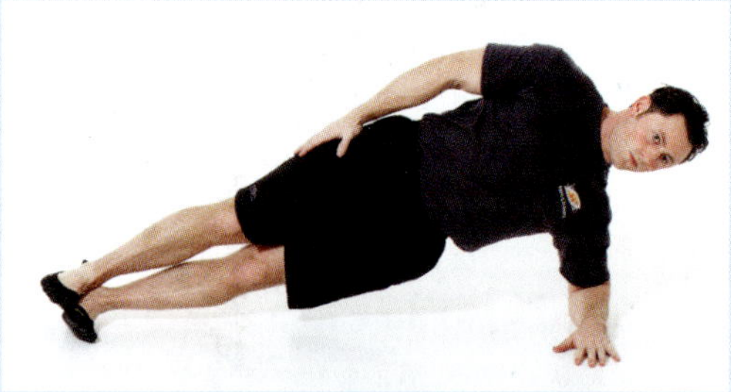

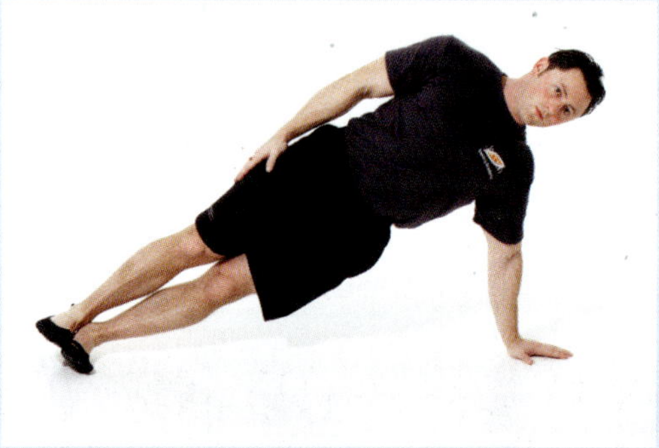

Execution
- Lie on the floor, on your side, with one foot in front of the other and the weight on the forearm.
- Lift the hips off the ground so that the body is in a straight line and hold this position.

FOUNDATION EXERCISES 9

There are a number of kettlebell exercises that provide the foundation techniques, skills and strength required to perform many of the advanced progressions and variations. These particular key or principle drills are almost always the first exercises taught to kettlebell enthusiasts (see table 9.1).

Table 9.1	Foundation kettlebell drills, in order of progression	
Order	Drill	Exercise number and page
1	Two hand swing	Exercise 5, page 57
2	One hand swing	Exercise 9, page 65
3	One hand (swing) snatch	Exercise 11, page 69
4	One hand (swing) clean	Exercise 16, page 76
5	One hand front squat	Exercise 17, page 79
6	One hand overhead press	Exercise 18, page 82
7	One hand Turkish get-up	Exercise 19, page 86
8	One hand windmill	Exercise 20, page 88

Even within this group of exercises there are still some drills that are taught before the others (see table 9.2).

Table 9.2	Foundation kettlebell drills by exercise
Type of exercise	Drills, by progression
Swing	Two hand swing, then one hand swing
Snatch	One hand swing, then one hand (swing) snatch
Clean	One hand swing, then rack position, one hand front squat and one hand (swing) clean
Press	One hand windmill, then rack position and one hand overhead press

When first learning the kettlebell foundation drills, undertake the following progressions: first, the two hand swing, one hand swing, rack position, one hand front squat, one hand windmill and one hand Turkish get-up. These will provide the key start position, partial techniques, range of motion or stability required to then apply to the following drills: the one hand (swing) snatch, one hand (swing) clean and one hand overhead press.

TWO HAND SWING

The kettlebell swing is a continuous, rhythmical drill where the kettlebell is taken from between the legs in an arc to a position at about shoulder height. The swing is the archetypal kettlebell exercise. If there is a single drill that is included in every kettlebell book, within every kettlebell instructor course, on every kettlebell website and has more YouTube videos than any other kettlebell exercise, it is the two hand kettlebell swing. It is the drill that provides the foundation technique for the one hand swing, the snatch and the clean and all of their progressions and variations. Because of this, there is more debate relating to its correct technique than with any other kettlebell exercise.

The swing was originally a strongman exercise, performed with a dumbbell and from a 'dead start' position on the floor. It was not a continuous, rhythmical exercise and was trained more like a set of individual or multiple deadlifts. The aim of the strongman dumbbell swing (dead start) was to teach the 'art of the flat back'. Today, we refer to this skill as the ability to maintain a neutral spine, and it is one of the first practical skills that fitness instructors and personal trainers learn in any course. The ability to differentiate between hip flexion (bending forward at the waist) and spinal flexion (rounding the back or curling forward) is crucial for practicing good technique for exercises such as the squat, deadlift or bent-over row.

Over the last hundred years or so the kettlebell swing has evolved into the continuous drill that many are familiar with today. The continuous swing can be performed with a dumbbell, medicine ball or even weight plate, but the kettlebell version is one of the most comfortable and effective. As the saying goes, a good workman uses the right tool for the right job, and the kettlebell is probably the best tool for the continuous swing.

The two hand kettlebell swing works the posterior chain muscles (the hamstrings on the back of the thighs, the erector spinae running up the back and even the calves to a lesser extent) as well as the posterior sling muscles (the latissimus dorsi, the large back muscle; the gluteus maximus, the muscles of the butt that extend the hips to a straight position and the fascia or sheath that links these muscles). These muscles work together to extend the hips from a flexed position; the same movement that occurs when you perform a vertical jump upwards or throw an object upwards and behind you. The bell swings between the legs and backwards to load the muscles by getting in a good 'lifting position' and the speed of the swing also stimulates the muscle spindles (see box).

ORDER OF PROGRESSION

The two hand kettlebell swing (exercise 5, page 57) is a lift pattern exercise that is performed ballistically (at a high velocity) and for sustained repetitions. To safely apply it within your exercise programme, you should master the following teaching progressions:

- Exercise 1 Two hand Romanian deadlift (RDL) with one kettlebell (page 55)
- Exercise 2 Two hand dead swing with one kettlebell (page 55)
- Exercise 3 Dead swing with fingers release, one kettlebell (page 56)
- Exercise 4 Two hand mini swings with one kettlebell (page 56)

Muscle spindles

Muscle spindles are a protective group of specialised muscle cells located in all muscles. Their role is to protect against muscles over-lengthening and/or tearing by sensing any lengthening of the muscle and at what speed this lengthening occurs. If stimulated, they cause a subsequent contraction of the muscle, which causes it to shorten. This is why we must perform dynamic stretching as part of the warm-up because this stimulates the muscle spindles and causes the nervous system to send 'contraction messages' to the muscles being worked in the session.

spine in a neutral position (slight curvature in the low back) or flat, but definitely not rounded. The shins should be vertical and there should be a reasonable degree of tension in the hamstrings and glutes.
- Take a small breath in and activate (brace) the core, then press through the floor and push the hips forward to lift the bell up to the hips.
- Pause briefly, then hinge the hips backwards and slowly reach between the legs and back to place the kettlebell into its original start position.

Exercise 2 Two hand RDL with one kettlebell

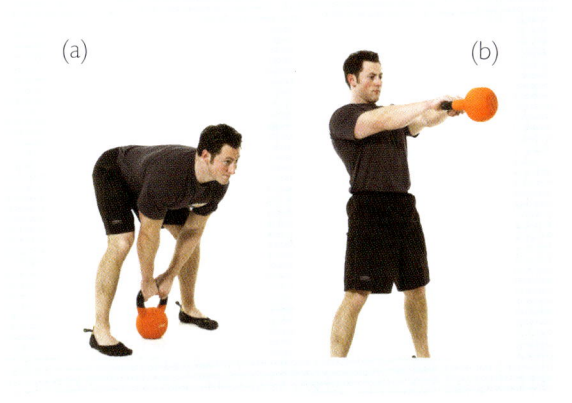

(a)   (b)

Exercise 1 Two hand RDL with one kettlebell

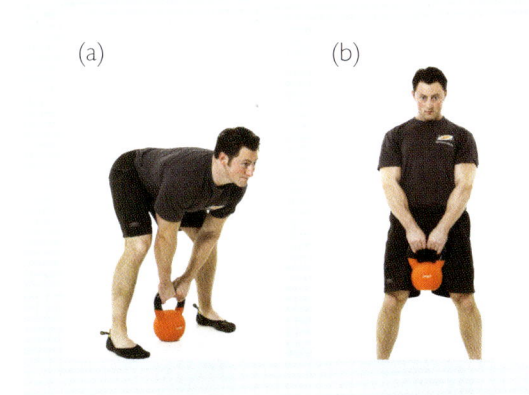

(a)   (b)

Execution
- Position the body with feet about shoulder width apart and the kettlebell facing forward at a position in line with the heels.
- Take hold of the handle with both hands and gently grip. The chest should be high with the

Execution
- Start in the same position as exercise 1 with the shins vertical and tension in the hamstrings and glutes.
- Take a small breath in and activate (brace) the core, then press through the floor and explosively push the hips forward to dynamically lift the bell upwards and forwards. In this mid-position the body should be upright, with the glutes maximally contracted and the spine neutral.

- The bell should be projected upwards anywhere between hip and chest height, with the arms extended and relaxed. The bell should not be lifted up with the upper body, but the force of the hip extension should project it upwards.
- Do not hold the bell in the top position. Allow the bell to swing back down, controlling it back to the start position between the feet.
- Hold the dead position for 1–3 seconds before starting the next repetition.

Exercise 3 Dead swing with finger release, one kettlebell

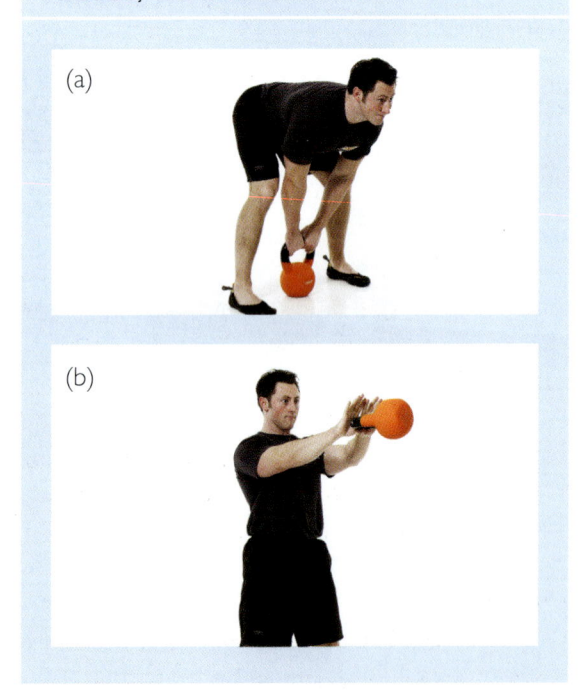

(a)

(b)

This is a great drill for anyone who lifts the bell up with their arms to correct that fault.

Execution
- Start in the same position as exercise 1 with the shins vertical and tension in the hamstrings and glutes.
- Take a small breath in and activate (brace) the core, then press through the floor and explosively push the hips forward to dynamically lift the bell upwards and forwards.
- As the bell is projected upwards to chest height, with the arms extended and relaxed, relax the grip on the handle and release the fingers briefly.
- As the bell is projected upwards it reaches the peak of its arc, where the kettlebell becomes weightless briefly (called 'the transition'). It is at this point where you should release the grip and, if timed correctly, the kettlebell should not move.
- As the bell drops, grip the handle again with the fingers and guide back to the start position.
- Hold the dead position for 1–3 seconds before starting the next repetition.

Exercise 4 Two hand mini swings with one kettlebell

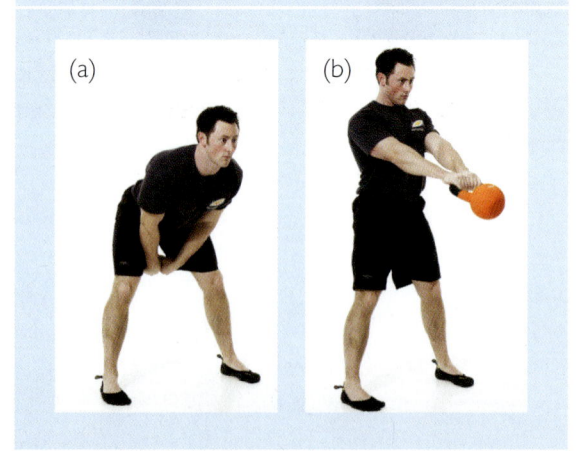

(a)   (b)

This drill is designed to teach the rhythmical nature of continuous swings and to learn when to relax as the bell becomes weightless, and when to exert to generate the force to project the bell upwards.

Execution
- Start in the same position as exercise 1 with the shins vertical and tension in the hamstrings and glutes.
- Take a small breath in and activate (brace) the core, then press through the floor and explosively push the hips forward to dynamically lift the bell upwards and forwards.
- As the bell become weightless and drops, guide it back between the legs to load the posterior chain and place the body in the deadlift position.
- As the bell becomes weightless again extend the hips forward to lift the bell up to about abdomen height. Do not try to reach to lift the bell all the way up to chest height or to reach too far back between the legs.
- Perform this drill for 20 seconds before resting and repeating.
- Do not perform this drill for too long so that technique falters or the muscles become fatigued; this is still predominantly a teaching drill.

Exercise 5 Two hand swing with one kettlebell

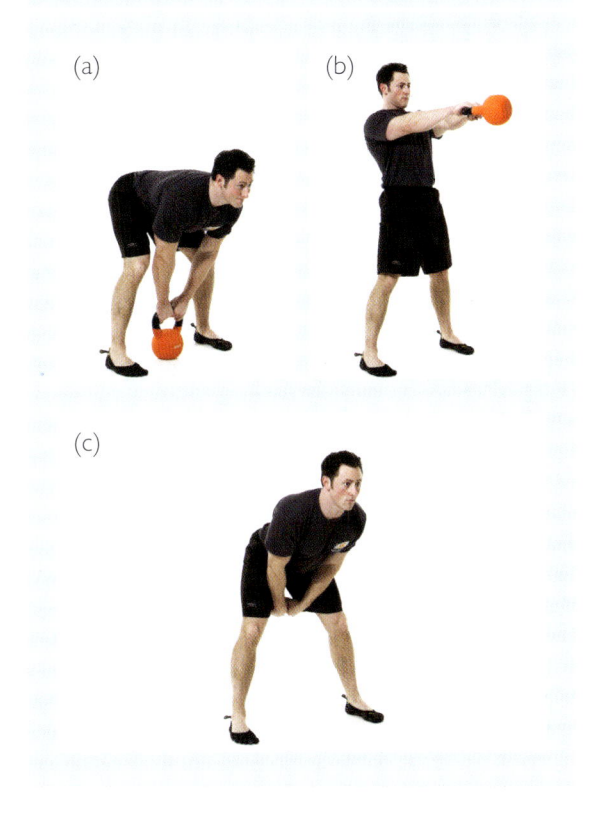

(a) (b)

(c)

Aims
The aims of this drill are to teach a ballistic lifting technique and to work the posterior (extensor) chain muscles in a lifting pattern.

Set-up
- Stand with feet approximately shoulder width apart or slightly wider.
- Keep your feet flat throughout the exercise and in a natural position, ideally at about 20–30 degrees from pointing forward.
- Position the kettlebell with the handle aligned between your heels.

- Bend forward from the hips, keeping the spine neutral, and grip the handle with both hands. The hips should go back, to keep the weight on the heels and mid-foot, and the upper torso should be near horizontal.
- Try to keep your shins vertical and limit knee bend; flexing or bending the knees recruits more of the quadriceps and diminishes the activation of the hamstrings and glutes at the back. It then becomes more of a squat (sitting) pattern, rather than the lifting pattern it should be.

Execution
- Take a breath in, hold it and brace your core muscles.
- Contract the muscles of the glutes and hamstrings to quickly bring the hips forward to a fully extended (upright) position. This movement should drive the kettlebell upwards towards about shoulder height.
- The muscles around the posterior hip are the muscles that lift the bell, transmitting the force when they contract through the core, shoulders and arms and into the kettlebell.
- The kettlebell should reach the peak of the arc of the swing at approximately chest or shoulder height. At this point the body position should look like an upside-down 'L', with the legs and upper torso in a vertical straight line and the arms forming the horizontal line. The kettlebell should be an extension of the arms, horizontal and flat at the top, where it becomes briefly weightless.
- As the kettlebell drops, guide it back towards the groin and between the legs, hinging the hips back. Keep the hands close to the groin, but avoid touching the forearms on the insides of the thighs.
- As the hands reach backwards and behind, getting into a similar 'lift position' as taken during the beginning of the drill, the kettlebell becomes weightless again.
- At this second transition point contract the glutes and hamstrings ballistically and repeat.

Key points
- Focus on keeping the glutes taut throughout each and every repetition.
- Keep the back flat or neutral; avoid rounding the back as you reach between the legs and avoid overarching the back when stood upright.
- The weight should be on your heels and mid-foot.
- The hips, core and arms should work as a single unit transmitting force efficiently through to the bell to lift it.
- Limit knee bend to effectively load and work the posterior chain and posterior sling muscles.
- The top position should look like an upside-down 'L'.
- The kettlebell should always be an extension of the arms, not flicking up or sagging during the swing.

Key errors
- Lifting the bell using the upper body (see figure 9.1). The bell will likely hang down from the handle throughout the concentric phase. To correct, focus on using the stronger hip extensors and posterior chain muscles and practise dead swings with finger release.
- The bell flips up at the beginning of the eccentric phase. This is due to the individual

not allowing the bell to drop by itself (at the speed of gravity), but trying to force it down. The individual pushes down on the handle while the bell is weightless thus causing the bell to flip upwards (seemingly).

- Stopping the bell on the concentric phase. The bell will likely flip upwards at the end of the concentric phase (see figure 9.2). This means that excessive force is being transferred to the bell and instead of it swinging above the head, the individual is deliberately stopping the bell at chest height, rather than it naturally stopping at this height. Less force is required; use only enough force to project the bell to chest height, or use a heavier bell that requires more force to lift it to that height.
- The bell hangs down at the top. If the bell follows a good position for the concentric phase but then hangs down at the top position, it usually means that the individual is holding this point (the point of transformation where the bell becomes weightless) for too long. Try to better feel the rhythm, allow gravity to drop the bell down and don't hold the isometric phase (at the end of the concentric phase) for too long.
- The bell is too far forward at the end of the concentric phase. This will likely cause insufficient extension, as the body will be slightly flexed at the hips as a result. The individual should try to keep the bell close throughout both phases, especially the concentric, by pulling the bell towards them and drawing back the shoulders into the sockets.

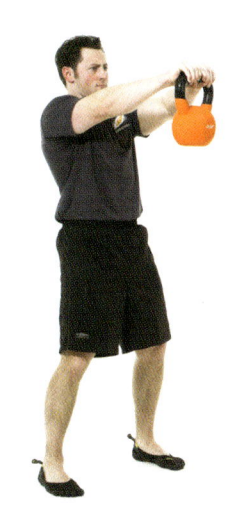

Figure 9.1 Do not lift the bell using the upper body.

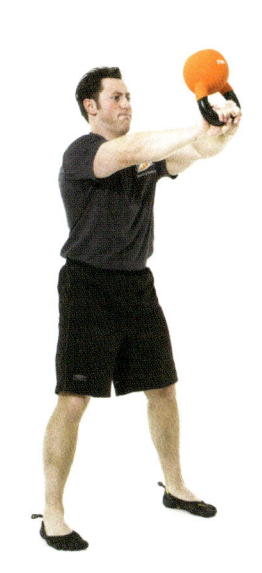

Figure 9.2 Avoid stopping the bell on the concentric phase.

- Full extension at the hips is not achieved (hips are flexed at top position). This may be due to poor bell trajectory, weak or inactive glutes or tight hip flexors. Undertake remedial drills to release the hip flexors and drills to activate the glutes and hamstrings, and then apply back into the swing exercise to test for improvement.
- The bell flips at the end of the eccentric phase (see figure 9.3). This can be due to being too upright through the torso or the forearms touching the inner thighs, or both. Because there is still momentum in the bell and the forearms cannot move, the bell continues its motion by flipping up towards the glutes/tailbone. To correct, lean a little further forward, and keep the forearms off the thighs.
- Rounding of the back (see figure 9.4). The individual needs to differentiate between hip flexion and spinal flexion, and practise hinging at the hips. Practise the regression drills to the swing – hip hinge, RDL, dead swing, mini swings.
- Being pulled forward (see figure 9.5). Whether this occurs on the concentric or eccentric phase, it is due to poor bell trajectory. Any significant transfer of weight shifting on to the toes is indicative of the bell coming too far forward. On the concentric phase, focus on transferring the force from the posterior chain to get the bell upwards rather than forwards. On the eccentric phase guide the bell back and between the legs.
- Heels lifting off the ground during the swing. It is usual for the heels to come off the ground during barbell snatches and cleans because of the force required for this single repetition. For repetitive swings, though, it is important to maintain a connection through the feet with the floor and to be grounded throughout the set.

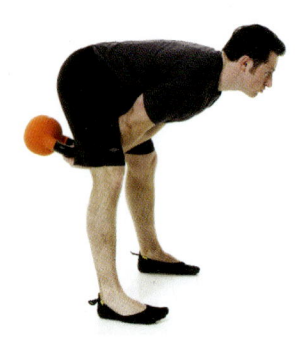

Figure 9.3 Don't allow the bell to flip at the end of the eccentric phase.

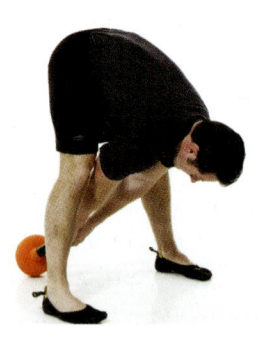

Figure 9.4 It is essential to avoid rounding the back.

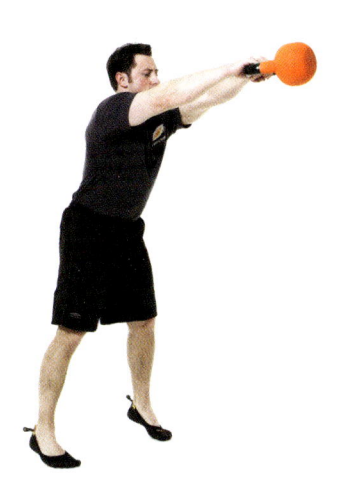

Figure 9.5 Do not allow the bell to pull you forwards.

- Being too upright in the torso/using the quads and not the hamstrings. If an individual naturally tends to squat down to perform the swings, and is not simply taught this way, then a few factors can be inferred from this. It is usually due to insufficient strength/strength-endurance in the posterior chain. This can be the result of a previous injury or just a lack of conditioning. They may squat to utilise the quads more and limit the loading on the lower back (an integral part of the posterior chain). If a client is weak in the posterior chain, this is a more efficient way for them to swing the bell. But they should look to improve posterior chain strength and mobility (hamstrings, glutes, low back). This may be better done with slow tempo resistance training (e.g. the RDL) as a regression to the kettlebell swing.
- Gripping the bell too tightly. Keep enough of a grip on the bell so that it doesn't slip out of your hands, but it should be able to move freely within the fingers.
- Leaning back at the top (see figure 9.6). Many individuals over-recruit the lower back muscles and lean back at the top of the swing. This is usually to compensate for weak glutes and insufficient hip extension force, so the spinal extensors try to generate the force instead.
- Kettlebell is too low on eccentric phase (see figure 9.7). The kettlebell should not be allowed to swing near the floor as the load on the back will be too great, making it more difficult to effectively activate the glutes and hamstrings. As soon as the bell becomes weightless at the top of the swing, guide it backwards towards the groin, making sure the hips are hinged backwards at the same time to move them out of the way.
- Flicking the kettlebell off the pelvis. The coaching cue 'use the hips' is taken a little too literally and the kettlebell is actually pushed up and off the front of the hips. Keep the arms off the hips and focus on more use of the posterior hip musculature.

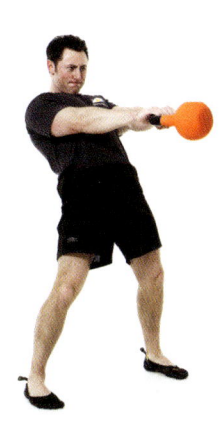

Figure 9.6 Avoid leaning back at the top of the phase.

FOUNDATION EXERCISES

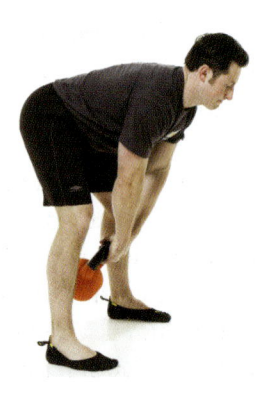

Figure 9.7 Ensure the kettlebell isn't too low during the eccentric phase.

Exercise variations
Rigid or hard style
The rigid style involves more emphasis on a strong hip extension, referred to as a 'hip snap', a forced expiration of air on the concentric phase, a tighter grip on the bell and more quadriceps involvement. It is usually performed in shorter sets.

Fluid style
The fluid style or Girevoy style (GS) involves more use of the elastic loading of the hip extensors by having the knees straighter, less active focus on snapping the hips to full extension, a looser grip and breathing in on the concentric phase. It has a generally more relaxed feel so that little effort is used, more energy is saved and the sets can continue for longer.

Additional notes
- Individuals should be able to lift some of the heaviest loads on a two hand swing in comparison with other kettlebell drills.
- Ensure you can perform the slow tempo variations of the prerequisite drills – RDL, dead swings, etc.
- Develop good posterior chain strength and endurance prior to using the kettlebell two hand swing.
- Vary the position slightly to find the optimal placement of hips, knees and the bell.
- Ensure the swing has a cyclical activity with a steady rhythm.
- Master the two hand swing before progressing to the one hand swing.
- Use the rigid style for short sets, with more strength emphasis, and the fluid style for longer sets, with more strength-endurance emphasis.
- For beginners it is commonly easier to teach the rigid method first and then adapt into the fluid style when appropriate.
- Include this exercise as a 'lifting pattern' drill within your training programme.
- Keep the reps low when learning the technique and gradually build up.

ONE HAND SWING
The one hand swing, also known as the single hand swing, is a progression from the two hand swing and is simply a single hand grip version of it. Virtually all of the teaching points and common errors are the same, and the prerequisite drills are similar to the two hand swing. The one hand swing is a crucial drill to learn as it forms part of the techniques required for the clean and the snatch.

ORDER OF PROGRESSION
The one hand swing (exercise 9, page 65) works the posterior chain muscles (the hamstrings and

the erector spinae) as well as the posterior sling muscles (the latissimus dorsi and the glutes). It is a lift pattern exercise that is performed ballistically and over sustained repetitions. To safely apply this exercise with your exercise programme you should master the following teaching regressions.

- Exercise 6 One hand dead swing with one kettlebell (this page)
- Exercise 7 One hand dead swing with finger release and one kettlebell (page 64)
- Exercise 8 One hand mini swings with one kettlebell (page 64)

Exercise 6 One hand dead swing with one kettlebell

(a)   (b)

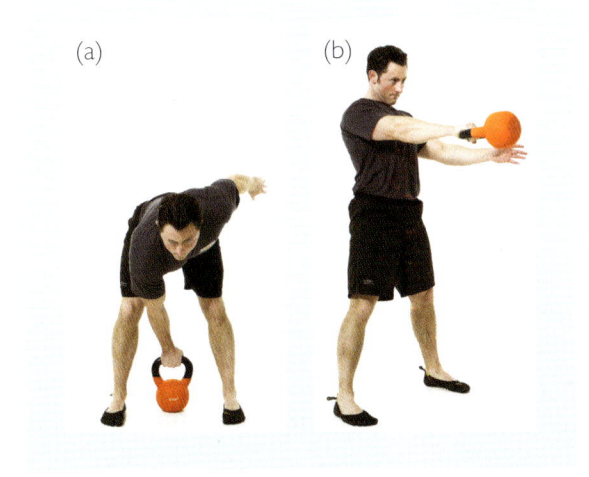

Execution
- Position the body with feet about shoulder width apart and the kettlebell facing forward on a position in line with the heels.
- Take hold of the handle with one hand and gently grip. The chest should be high with the spine in a neutral position or flat. The shins should be vertical and there should be a reasonable degree of tension in the hamstrings and glutes.
- Take a small breath in and activate (brace) the core, then press through the floor and explosively push the hips forward to dynamically lift the bell upwards and forwards.
- In this mid-position the body should be upright, with the glutes maximally contracted and the spine neutral. The bell should be projected upwards anywhere between hip and chest height, with the arm extended and relaxed. The bell should not be lifted up with the upper body, but the force of the hip extension should project it upwards.
- Allow the bell to swing back down, control it back to the start position between the feet and hold the dead position for 1–3 seconds before starting the next repetition.

FOUNDATION EXERCISES

Exercise 7 One hand dead swing with with finger release and one kettlebell

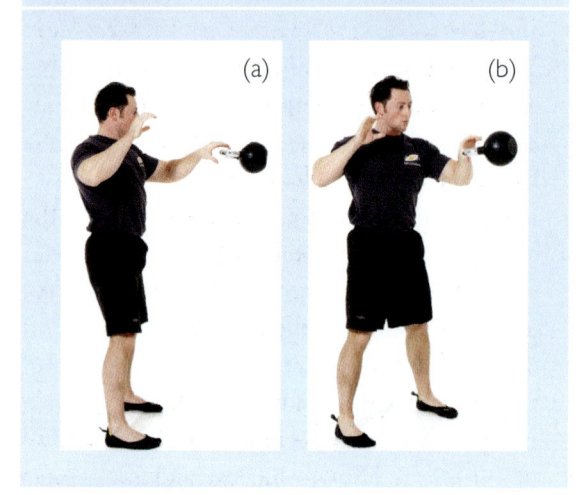

(a) (b)

Exercise 8 One hand mini swings with one kettlebell

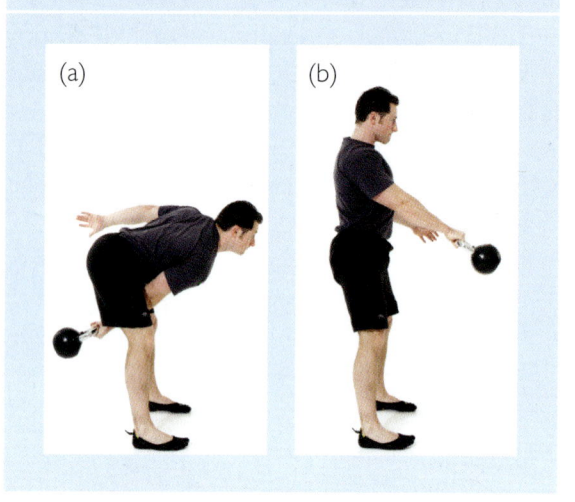

(a) (b)

Execution
- Start in the same position as exercise 6 with the shins vertical and tension in the hamstrings and glutes.
- Take a small breath in and activate (brace) the core, then press through the floor and explosively push the hips forward to dynamically lift the bell upwards and forwards.
- As the bell is projected upwards to chest height, with the arm extended and relaxed, relax the grip on the handle and release the fingers briefly.
- Again, if timed correctly the kettlebell should not move.
- As the bell drops, grip the handle again with the fingers and guide back to the start position.
- Hold the dead position for 1–3 seconds before starting the next repetition.

Execution
- Start in the same position as exercise 6 with the shins vertical and tension in the hamstrings and glutes.
- Take a small breath in and activate (brace) the core, then press through the floor and explosively push the hips forward to dynamically lift the bell upwards and forwards.
- As the bell become weightless and drops, guide it back between the legs to load the posterior chain and place the body in the deadlift position.
- As the bell becomes weightless again, extend the hips forward to lift the bell up to about abdomen height.
- Perform for sets of about 20–30 seconds.

Exercise 9 One hand swing

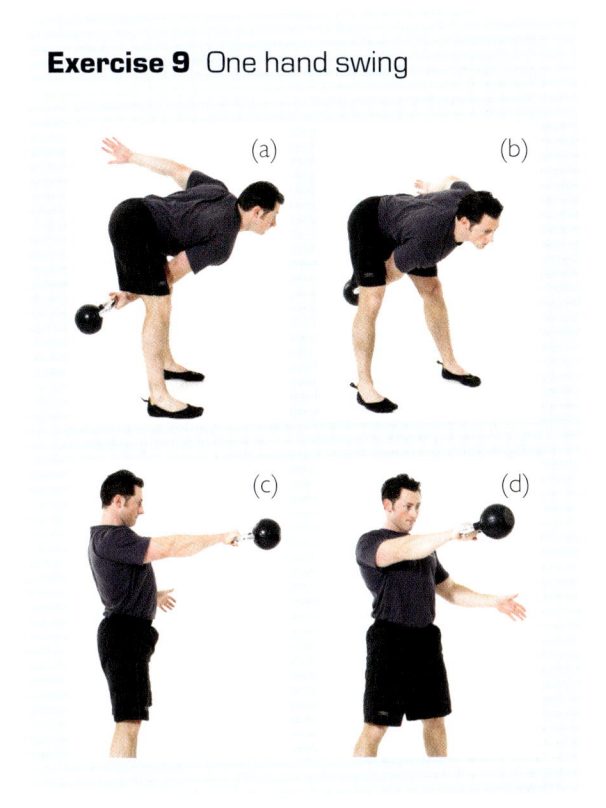

(a) (b) (c) (d)

Aims

The aim of the one hand kettlebell swing is to progress from the two hand swing and to work the posterior (extensor) chain muscles in a unilateral lifting pattern.

Set-up

- Position the body with feet about shoulder width apart and the kettlebell facing forward in line with the heels.
- Take hold of the handle with one hand and gently grip. The chest should be high with the spine in a neutral position or flat. The shins should be vertical and there should be a reasonable degree of tension in the hamstrings and glutes.

Execution

- Take a breath in, hold it and brace your core muscles.
- Contract the muscles of the glutes and hamstrings to quickly bring the hips forward to a fully extended (upright) position. This movement should drive the kettlebell upwards towards about shoulder height.
- Ensure the posterior hip muscles are the muscles that lift the bell, transmitting the force when they contract through the core, shoulders and arms and into the kettlebell.
- The kettlebell should reach the peak of the arc of the swing at approximately shoulder height. At this point the body position should look like an upside-down 'L', with the legs and upper torso in a vertical straight line and the arm forming the horizontal line. The kettlebell should be an extension of the arm, horizontal and flat at the top, where it becomes briefly weightless.
- As the kettlebell drops, guide it back towards the groin and between the legs, hinging the hips back. Keep the hand close to the groin, but avoid touching the forearm on the insides of the thighs.
- As the hand reaches backwards and behind, getting into a similar 'lift position' as at the beginning of the drill, the kettlebell becomes weightless again.
- Contract the glutes and hamstrings and repeat.
- Use the other arm to help generate force with the hips, just as you would when performing a vertical jump.
- As the hand holding the kettlebell reaches between the legs, the other arm should be reaching back as well (see exercise 9a). As the hips extend, this arm comes forward to level with the body.

FOUNDATION EXERCISES

Key points

- Focus on keeping the glutes taut throughout each and every repetition.
- Keep the back flat or neutral; avoid rounding the back as you reach between your legs and/or overarching it when stood upright.
- The weight should be on your heels and mid-foot.
- Use the hips, core and arms as a single unit transmitting force efficiently through to the bell to lift it.
- Limit knee bend to effectively load and work the posterior chain and posterior sling muscles.
- The top position should look like an upside-down 'L'.
- Pivot at the hips.
- Draw the shoulder back into the socket when lifting the kettlebell.
- The bell should extend out as a continuation of the arm.

Key errors

- The bell is too far forward at the end of the concentric phase. This will likely cause insufficient extension, as the body will be slightly flexed at the hips as a result. Try to keep the bell close throughout both phases, especially the concentric, by pulling the bell towards you and sucking the shoulder into the socket.
- The bell flips at the end of the eccentric phase. This is usually due to being too upright through the torso and the forearm touching the inner thighs. Because there is still momentum in the bell and the forearm cannot move, the bell continues its motion by flipping up towards the glutes/tailbone.
- Rounding of the back. You need to differentiate between hip flexion and spinal flexion and practise hinging at the hips. You will drop the shoulder more on the one hand swing to stretch the lat and load the contralateral glute better.
- Being pulled forward. Whether this occurs on the concentric or eccentric phases, it is due to poor bell trajectory. Any significant transfer of weight shifting on to the toes is indicative of the bell coming too far forward. On the concentric phase, focus on transferring the force from the posterior chain to get the bell upwards, rather than forwards. On the eccentric phase, guide the bell back and between the legs.
- Being too upright in the torso/using the quads and not the hamstrings. Look to improve posterior chain strength and mobility (hamstrings, glutes, lower back). This may be better done with slow tempo resistance training (RDL) as a regression to the swing.
- Gripping the bell too tightly. Keep enough of a grip on the bell so that it doesn't slip out of your hands, but it should be able to move freely within the fingers.
- Leaning back at top. Many individuals over-recruit the lower back muscles and lean back at the top of the swing. This is usually to compensate for weak glutes and insufficient hip extension force, so the spinal extensors try to generate the force instead.
- Rotating too much. As the hand reaches between the legs, the shoulder rolls more than during the two hand swing and if this is not controlled it can cause pronation and supination patterns in the legs, as seen by the knees caving in or out, depending on which side it is. Focus on controlling the shoulder roll and not allowing it to negatively affect the lower body mechanics.

Additional notes

- The load for the one hand swing is lighter than the two hand swing.
- Develop good posterior chain strength and endurance prior to using the one hand swing.
- Vary your position slightly to find the optimal placement of hips, knees and bell.
- It should be a cyclical activity with a steady rhythm.
- Master the two hand swing before progressing to the one hand swing.
- Master the one hand swing before progressing to the one hand snatch.
- Use the rigid style for short sets, with more strength emphasis, and fluid style for longer sets, with more strength-endurance emphasis.
- For beginners, it is commonly easier to teach the rigid method first and then adapt into the fluid style when appropriate.
- Play around with the hand position to see what feels most comfortable. Some prefer to keep the hand pronated throughout, while others keep the thumb pointing down when swinging between the legs and pronated at the top. A few like to have the hand semi-supinated throughout with the thumb pointing upwards.
- Use as a 'lifting pattern' exercise within your training programme.

ONE HAND (SWING) SNATCH

The snatch is an exercise where the load, in this case the kettlebell, is taken from the floor or a position beneath the hips to a position above the head in a single motion. The snatch involves three phases: a lift phase, using the hip extensors (glutes and hamstrings); an upward pull phase, using the upper back, shoulders and biceps; and the punch or catch phase. The lift phase may be from a dead start position or from a swing, but it engages the muscles involved in hip extension (glutes, hamstrings, latissimus dorsi and the erector spinae working isometrically). These lifting muscles, work synergistically with the pulling muscles, projecting the bell up to a position above the head. The glutes and hamstrings get the bell moving upwards, while the upward pull of the back, biceps and shoulders directs the bell vertically upwards. The upper and lower body need to work together efficiently or the bell will not reach the required height.

After the lift phase and the pull phase, the final phase is the punch or the catch phase, where the handle is rotated around the bell, so that the bell 'rolls' into the finish position above the head. As soon as the bell has been pulled upwards, close to the body with the elbow lifting up and slightly out, the lifting hand (gripped around the handle) punches forwards and upwards. This final movement needs to be timed perfectly so that as the bell reaches the peak of its arc and starts to slow and become weightless, the handle is rotated underneath the bell so that it lands gently on the forearm of the lifting arm.

ORDER OF PROGRESSION

The one hand snatch, which is sometimes called the swing snatch, is a progression from the one hand swing and involves an additional upwards pull phase, more aggression and more force development. The term 'swing snatch' can be used to describe the fact that the bell is swung between the legs with each repetition rather than being lifted from a stop position on the floor, which is referred to as a 'dead snatch'.

The one hand (swing) snatch (exercise 11, page 69) is a lift and pull pattern exercise that is performed ballistically and for sustained repetitions. In kettlebell competitions, the one hand kettlebell snatch is performed for 10 minutes (5 minutes each arm) to see how many repetitions can be achieved in that time. To safely apply this drill within your exercise programme you should master the following teaching progressions:

- Exercise 9 One hand swing with one kettlebell (page 65)
- Exercise 10 One hand high pulls with one kettlebell (page 68)

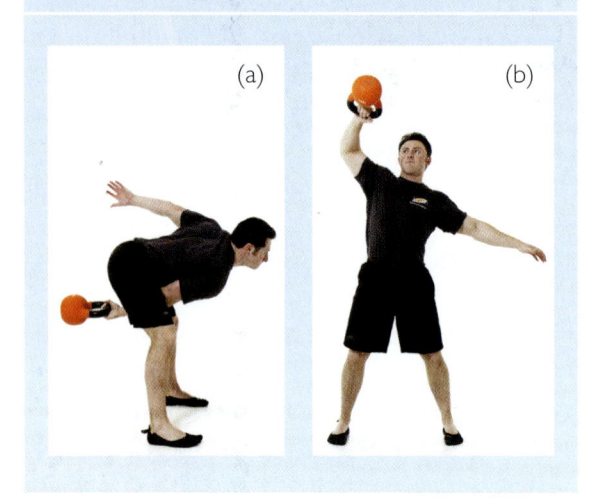

Exercise 10 One hand high pulls with one kettlebell

(a)   (b)

Execution
- Position the body with feet about shoulder width apart and the kettlebell facing forward in line with the heels.
- Take hold of the handle with one hand and gently grip. The chest should be high with the spine in a neutral position or flat. The shins should be vertical and there should be a reasonable degree of tension in the hamstrings and glutes.
- Take a small breath in and activate (brace) the core, then perform a dead swing. Let the bell swing between the legs and then perform the same concentric phase of a swing, but this time initiate a strong upright pull as the bell moves forward of the hips. The bell should be projected upwards to about head height or above, with the arm bent at the elbow.
- As the bell becomes weightless, follow it downwards and guide it between the legs, as with the swing, and repeat.

Exercise 11 One hand (swing) snatch with one kettlebell

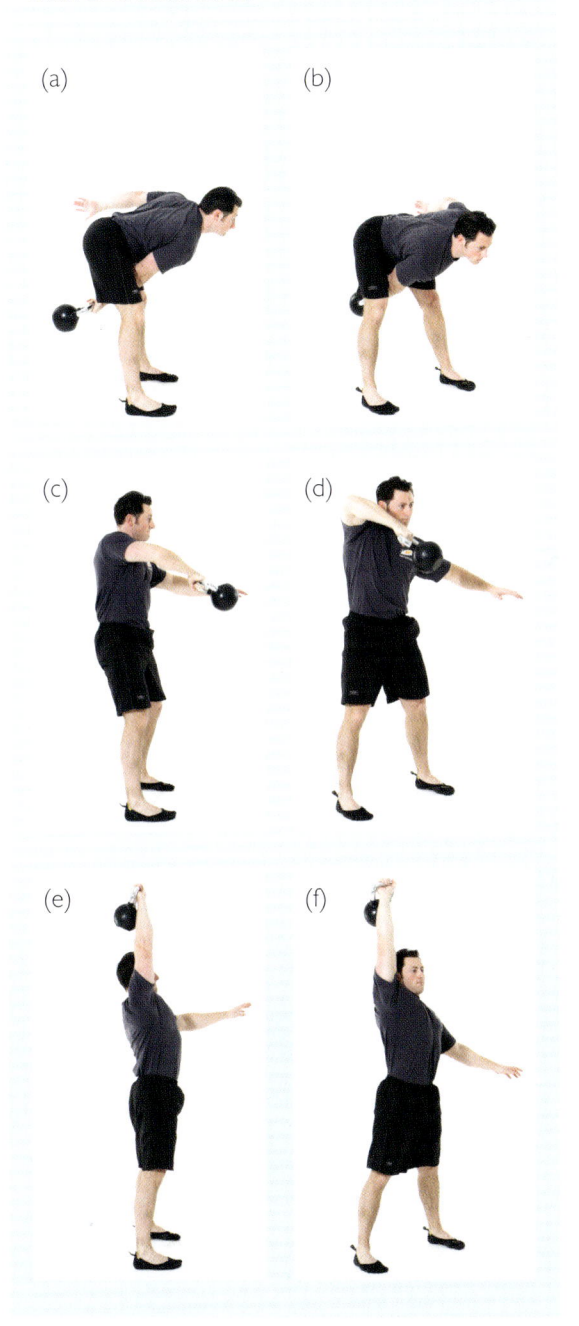

(a) (b)
(c) (d)
(e) (f)

Aims

The aims of the one hand (swing) snatch are to teach a ballistic lifting and upward pulling technique; to work the posterior (extensor) chain muscles, the pulling muscles of the shoulders, biceps and upper back, in a lifting and upward pulling pattern; to master the technique of lifting a weight above the head in a single action and to develop the correct technique required for events in the sport of kettlebell lifting.

Set-up

- Position the body with feet about shoulder width apart and the kettlebell facing forward in line with the heels.
- Take hold of the handle with one hand and gently grip. The chest should be high with the spine in a neutral position or flat. The shins should be vertical and there should be a reasonable degree of tension in the hamstrings and glutes.

Execution

- Perform one or two of the one hand swings to initiate the snatch, rather than trying to lift it above the head straight from the floor.
- As the bell falls from the peak of the swing, push the hips backwards, so that the kettlebell swings between the legs.
- As the bell becomes weightless forcefully extend the hips and knees to create the force to elevate the bell. The effort for the snatch should be twice as aggressive as for the one hand swing.
- As the bell moves forward of the hips as part of the swing, pull upwards and backwards on the kettlebell as if starting a lawnmower.
- As the bell accelerates upwards, punch upwards and forwards to flip the handle under the bell.

- In the finish catch position, the bell should rest on the forearm with the arm extended above the head.
- Drop the elbow and rotate the forearm so that the thumb rotates outwards and the bell rolls off the forearm and into the standard one hand swing grip.
- Guide the bell through the legs to load the hips for the next snatch repetition and repeat.

Key points
- Follow a fast 1-2-3 pattern – hips, pull, punch.
- Be very aggressive from the start of the concentric phase when the bell is between your legs.
- Pull the bell close to the body.
- Punch quickly upwards and with a small range of motion.

Key errors
- Too slow at the bottom. You need to be very aggressive with the movement of the hips to generate sufficient height with the kettlebell so it reaches the correct position for the punch. If you consider how much force you need to swing that weight, then think that for the snatch you need to get it higher (above the head) and faster for optimal technique.
- Too slow in the middle. You need to continue to accelerate the bell upwards, after the hip extension with a strong pull upwards. Without the powerful and fast bottom and middle phases of the snatch, the bell will not reach sufficient height above the head for the optimal 'catch' position to be achieved.
- Too slow at the top. As the bell reaches its maximum height of the pull, the idea is to rotate the handle around the bell so that it rests on the forearm in the catch position. The bell is only very briefly weightless, so the 'punch' phase of the snatch needs to be completed very quickly.
- Bell too far forward during snatch. The bell trajectory for the (swing) snatch is much closer and more vertical than the one hand swing. If the bell is too far forward, then when it is pulled back for the punch phase, there will be a significant impact on the forearm. It will also likely result in the bell being positioned too far forward in the catch position.
- No punch. Many individuals when learning the snatch undertake a fast lift and pull action, but without the 'punch' phase of rotating the handle around the bell, the bell will just flip over and fall downwards and backwards, resulting in significant contact with the forearm. There should be a fast pull-to-punch phase (see figure 9.8).
- Bell too far forward at the end position (see figure 9.9). At the top of the movement the elbow should be locked with the arm extended close to the ear and the handle positioned over the shoulder, hips and knee from both the front and the side views.

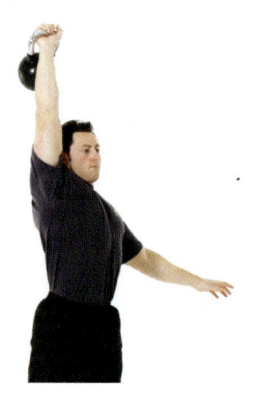

Figure 9.8 No punch will result in too much contact with the forearm.

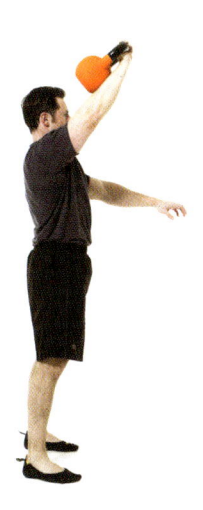

Figure 9.9 Don't let the bell fall too far forward at the end position.

- Casting the bell forward on the eccentric phase. Flicking the bell over and casting the bell forward disrupts the control of the eccentric phase, shifting the weight forward on to the toes and making it difficult to load the body effectively for the next repetition. Lower the kettlebell by dropping the elbow downwards, close to the body, thus discouraging casting forward.
- Poor timing of the extend-pull-punch phases. Each phase needs to integrate with the phase before and after for maximum force to get the bell into position to rotate the handle around it.
- Banging the kettlebell against the forearm. Although it takes practice to master the timing of the snatch, the bell should not bang against the forearm. Reasons for the bell banging against the forearm include being too slow at the top, the bell trajectory being too far forward, no 'punch' phase, or just poor timing of the extend-pull-punch phases.
- Rounding of the back. The individual needs to differentiate between hip flexion and spinal flexion, and practise hinging at the hips. You will drop the shoulder and reach more on the one hand snatch to stretch the lat and load the contralateral glute better to help generate more force.
- Gripping the bell too tightly. Keep enough of a grip on the bell so that it doesn't slip out of your hands, but it should be able to move freely within the fingers, even more so with the snatch than the swing.
- Not being aggressive enough. There are no passive movements in this drill until the kettlebell is locked at the top of the movement. Be aggressive as soon as the bell becomes weightless at the end of the eccentric phase as you reach between the legs.
- Squatting down as the bell goes between the legs rather than bending over. Being too upright in the torso can indicate that the quadriceps are being recruited and not the hamstrings and posterior chain muscles. To correct this fault look to improve posterior chain strength and mobility (hamstrings, glutes, low back). This is better done by regressing back to the swing or high pull.
- Cocked wrist at the top position (see figure 9.10). The wrist should be rigid and straight at the end of the concentric phase. If the bell sits in between the condyles of the wrist and is uncomfortable, then use a different design bell or wear a sweatband.
- The kettlebell swings too low to the ground. This is commonly due to casting the bell too far forward at the start of the concentric phase. It becomes difficult to control and too much energy is wasted slowing the bell down before it hits the floor.

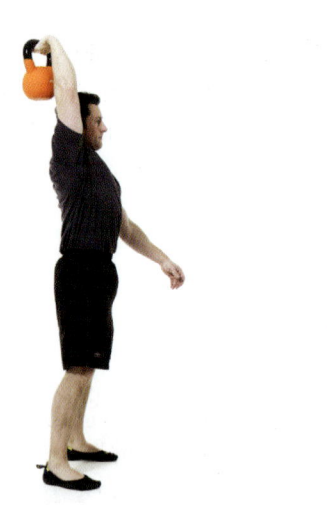

Figure 9.10 Do not cock the wrist at the top – it should be rigid and straight.

Additional notes

- The load for the one hand snatch is about the same as, or slightly lighter than, the one hand swing.
- Develop good posterior chain strength and endurance prior to using the one hand snatch.
- Vary your position slightly to find the optimal placement of hips, knees and bell.
- Treat each snatch as a separate lift or repetition. Make sure you pause between each rep – release the grip and hold the arm extended for a second or two before undertaking the next rep.
- Master the one hand swing and high pull before progressing to the one hand snatch.
- Use the rigid style for short sets, with more strength emphasis, and more fluid style for longer sets, with more strength-endurance emphasis.
- For beginners, it is commonly easier to teach the rigid method first and then adapt into the fluid style when appropriate.
- Use as an integrated 'lifting-pulling pattern' exercise within your training programme.

Exercise variations
Half snatch

When first learning the one hand snatch, it may be easier to start off with a half snatch. The half snatch is essentially the same technique as the swing snatch described above, but instead of performing the full eccentric phase, the kettlebell is lowered to the rack position on the chest then cast off into a swing between the legs. This is a good variation for many, in order to practise the concentric phase of the snatch without having to have perfected the eccentric phase. If the eccentric phase is not performed correctly, then a lot of energy is wasted and it makes the following concentric phase of the next repetition more difficult. As the bell swings between the legs this elastic energy is used to help generate the force to propel the bell above the head. Without this elastic energy, all of the force must come from the lifting and pulling muscles alone, making the exercise more difficult. It is the same when performing a vertical jump and pausing in the squat position for a few seconds, or holding the bar on the chest for three seconds during a bench press. The subsequent vertical jump is lower and it will be harder to lift the barbell on the bench press as a result of these pauses. Once the concentric, lifting phase of the swing snatch is perfected, then the eccentric phase can then be integrated into it.

Alternating swing snatch

An alternative to the half snatch is the alternating swing snatch. In between every repetition of the snatch a single repetition of a one hand swing is performed. The individual performs a swing-snatch-swing-snatch-swing and so on. Even if the lowering phase of the snatch isn't quite perfect, it won't affect the quality of the next repetition. The elastic energy from the swing provides the efficient build-up of elastic energy for the proceeding snatch.

Girevoy style (GS)

The punching phase of the snatch can be performed in a couple of ways. The first method is how many trainers teach it, while the second is more of a Girevoy (or competitive) style because it is slightly more efficient. The first method involves punching straight up, so that the handle rotates underneath the bell as it reaches the peak of its height. This technique is easy to explain and, for most, is easier to master. The downside is that it expends slightly more energy and the bell is required to be lifted marginally higher.

GS involves rotating the handle around the bell rather than underneath it (see figure 9.11). As the bell is pulled upwards, the hand is pulled inwards and upwards, which causes the handle to rotate around the bell rather than underneath, and causes the bell to 'roll' over the side of the forearm into the correct finishing position. This technique is much more energy efficient, hence it being the method of choice for kettlebell sport competitors.

Interestingly enough, when tutoring new trainers in the snatch exercise a large proportion out of 10 naturally, and without prompting, adopt this 'style' of completing the snatch – despite being prompted to punch underneath the bell and upwards – because it 'feels' easier to them. The other interesting fact is that it is pretty much the exact same technique used to lower the bell during the snatch, but done in reverse.

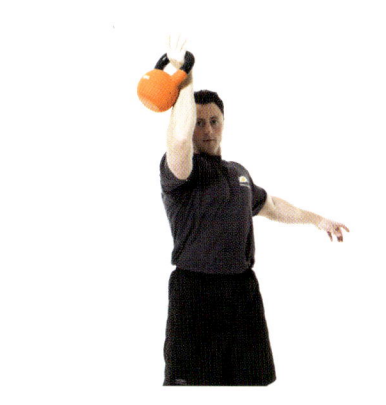

Figure 9.11 Girevoy style kettlebell snatch

ONE HAND (SWING) CLEAN

The clean involves three phases, as with the snatch: a lift phase, using the hip extensors (glutes and hamstrings); an upward pull phase, using the back, shoulders and biceps; and the punch or catch phase, where the bell is taken into the rack.

The lift phase may be from a dead start position or from a swing, but engages the muscles involved in hip extension (glutes, hamstrings, latissimus dorsi and the erector spinae working isometrically). These muscles provide the initial and majority of the force to get the bell to abdomen height.

As the bell is moving upwards and outwards in an arc, the pulling muscles of the upper body (deltoids, upper trapezius and biceps) redirect the bell vertically towards the optimal catch (rack) position. The upper and lower body should be working together as an efficient and coordinated unit; the lower body providing the force, with the upper body utilising this force and redirecting the bell trajectory.

The final phase is the punch or the catch phase, where the handle is rotated around the bell, so that the bell 'rolls' into the rack position. As soon as the bell has been pulled upwards, the bell should be close with the elbow lifting up and slightly out, and the lifting hand (gripped around the handle) punching inwards and upwards as if attempting to uppercut your own chin. This movement should get the elbow underneath the bell and next to (or just above) the hip. The motion of the hand could be described as a lift upwards, followed by a half clockwise stir – as if one were stirring a really big spoon for half a turn.

ORDER OF PROGRESSION

The one hand kettlebell (swing) clean (exercise 16, page 76) is a lift and pull pattern exercise that is performed ballistically and either for sustained repetitions, or to get the kettlebell into the rack position for the jerk, press or squat exercises, to name but a few. To safely apply this exercise with your exercise programme you should master the following teaching progressions.

- Exercise 9 One hand swing (page 65)
- Exercise 12 Rack position (page 74)
- Exercise 13 Two hand dead clean with one kettlebell (page 75)
- Exercise 14 One hand assisted dead clean with one kettlebell (page 75)
- Exercise 15 One hand dead clean with one kettlebell (page 75)

Exercise 12 Rack position

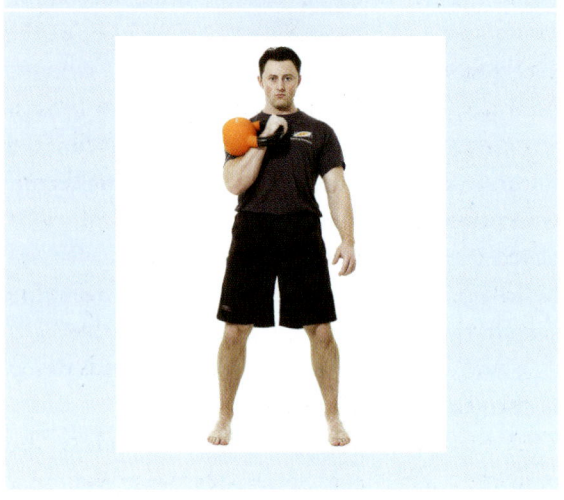

The rack is described as a position where the load is supported on or approximately at the chest and shoulders. It is a pausing position when taking the load, in this case the kettlebell, from the floor or a position beneath the hips to a position above the head in two stages. The clean exercise is the first stage, where the load is taken into the rack position.

Execution

- Grip the handle, with the knuckle of the thumb on the pec (chest muscle), the elbow close to the side, near the hip and the kettlebell resting on the forearm and the bicep.

Exercise 13 Two hand dead clean with one kettlebell

Execution
- With the kettlebell positioned sideways on, between the heels, take hold of the bell from both sides with both hands. The chest should be high, the shins should be vertical, with tension in the hamstrings and glutes.
- Take a small breath in and activate (brace) the core, then press through the floor and explosively push the hips forward and with two hands lifting the kettlebell into the rack position.
- Hold briefly then lower the kettlebell to the start position between the feet and repeat.

Exercise 14 One hand assisted dead clean with one kettlebell

Execution
- With the kettlebell positioned with the handle facing forward between the heels, take hold with one hand. The chest should be high; the shins should be vertical, with tension in the hamstrings and glutes.
- Take a small breath in and activate (brace) the core, then press through the floor and explosively push the hips forward and pull with the arm to lift the kettlebell.
- The other hand cups the bell during the pull to guide it into the correct rack position.
- Hold briefly, then lower the kettlebell to the start position between the feet and repeat.

Exercise 15 One hand dead clean with one kettlebell

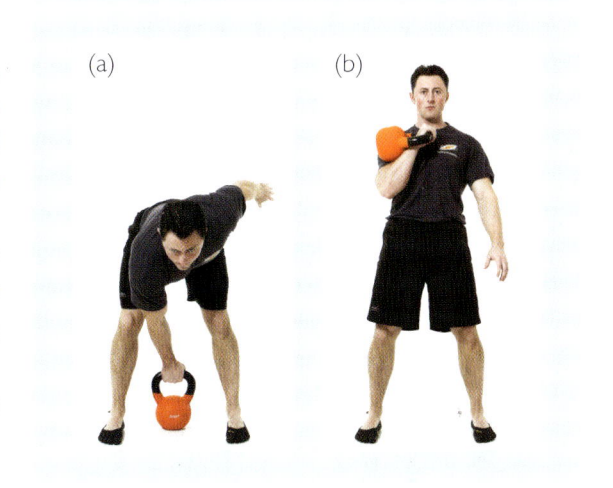

(a)   (b)

Execution
- Position the body with feet about shoulder width apart and the kettlebell facing forward in line with the heels.
- Take hold of the handle with one hand and gently grip. The chest should be high with the spine in a neutral position (slight curvature in the low back) or flat, but not rounded. The shins should be vertical and there should be a reasonable degree of tension in the hamstrings and glutes.
- Take a small breath in and activate (brace) the core, then press through the floor and explosively push the hips forward to dynamically lift the bell upwards, focusing on contracting the glutes and pull upwards with the arm.
- As the bell gets to just over hip height, punch the handle upwards and inwards as if trying to uppercut your own chin. This should cause the bell to 'roll' over the forearm into the finishing rack position. The elbow should be close to the body and just above the front of the hip.

- Hold briefly, then with either one or two hands (easier) lower the kettlebell to the start position between the feet and hold the dead position for 1–3 seconds before starting the next repetition.

Exercise 16 One hand (swing) clean with one kettlebell

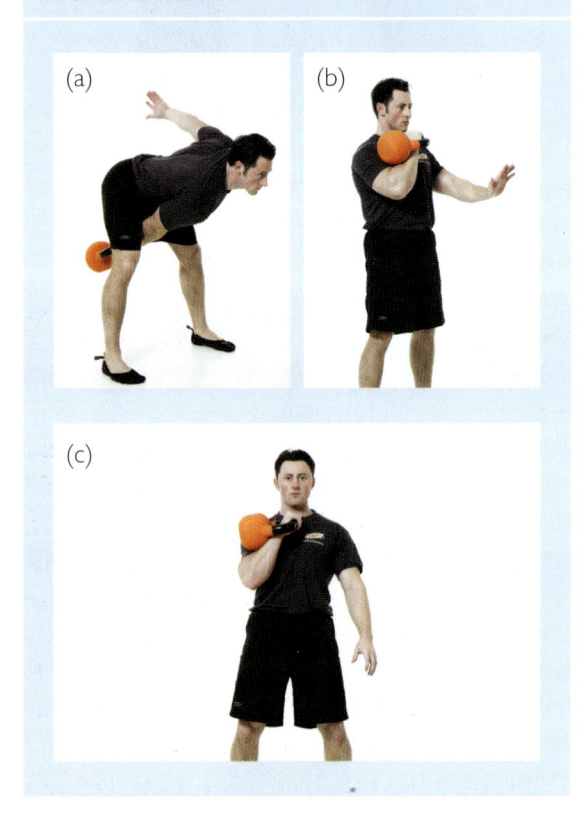

(a) (b) (c)

Aims

The aims of the one hand (swing) clean are to teach a ballistic lifting and upward pulling technique; to work the posterior (extensor) chain muscles, the pulling muscles of the shoulders, biceps and upper back in a lifting and upward pulling pattern; to master the technique of lifting a weight to the chest, or rack position, in a single action; and to develop the correct technique required for events in the sport of kettlebell lifting.

Set-up
- Position the body with feet about shoulder width apart and the kettlebell facing forward in line with the heels.
- Take hold of the handle with one hand and gently grip. The chest should be high with the spine in a neutral position or flat. The shins should be vertical and there should be a reasonable degree of tension in the hamstrings and glutes.

Execution
- Perform a dead clean (exercise 15, page 75) to get the kettlebell to the rack position.
- Roll the thumb forwards and allow the bell to drop forward, push the hips backwards, so that the kettlebell swings between the legs.
- As the bell becomes weightless at the transition point, forcefully extend the hips and knees to create the power to elevate the bell.
- As the bell moves forward of the hips as part of the swing, pull upwards and backwards on the kettlebell. As soon as the pull has been initiated, punch upwards, towards the chin, to flip the handle around the bell so that it rolls onto the forearm.
- In the rack position, the bell should rest on the forearm with the arm bent and the forearm diagonal across the chest and the fist on the same side pec. Hold this position for 1–2 seconds.
- Rotate the thumb forwards, so that the bell rolls off of the forearm and drops into the standard one hand swing grip. Guide the bell

through the legs, to load the hips for the next clean repetition and repeat.

- The effort for the clean should be less than that for the snatch because of the smaller distance required for it to travel. This usually means that a heavier kettlebell can be used.

Key points

- Follow a 1-2-3 pattern – hips, pull, uppercut punch.
- Use the momentum from the swing phase for power to lift the bell, then the force of the upwards pull to direct it upwards.
- Don't use just the upper body to lift the bell.
- Focus on getting the elbow underneath the bell quickly and on to the hip.

Key errors

- Bell too far forward during swing phase. The bell trajectory for the clean is much closer and more vertical than the one hand swing. If the bell is too far forward, then when it is pulled back for the catch in the rack position there will be a significant impact on the arm and shoulder. For athletes that require contact (martial artists, rugby players), this may be an acceptable adaptation to the exercise.
- No uppercut. Many individuals when learning the clean undertake a fast lift and pull action, but without the correct 'uppercut' phase of rotating the handle around the bell. The bell falls downwards resulting in significant contact with the forearm.
- Bell too far to the side at the rack position (see figure 9.12). At the rack position, the elbow should be locked into the side with the arm extended across the chest. Focus on pulling upwards rather than diagonally outwards to ensure correct positioning for the bell in the rack position.

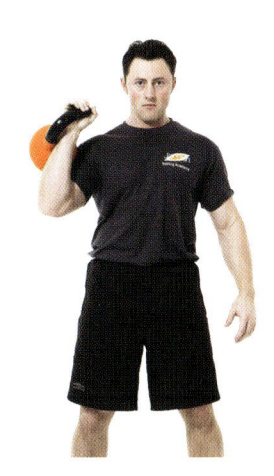

Figure 9.12 No uppercut means the bell lands on the forearm. Keep the elbow locked into the side.

- Casting the bell too far forward on the eccentric phase. Flicking the bell over and casting the bell too far forward will disrupt the control of the eccentric phase, shifting the weight forward on to the toes and making it difficult to load the body effectively for the next repetition. Lower the kettlebell by rotating the thumb forwards, dropping the kettlebell close to the body, thus discouraging casting forward.
- Banging the kettlebell against the forearm. Although it takes practice to master the timing of the clean, the bell should not bang against the forearm. Reasons for the bell banging against the forearm include being too slow with the uppercut, lifting the kettlebell too high or swinging the kettlebell too far forward on the upward phase.

- Rounding of the back. The individual needs to differentiate between hip flexion and spinal flexion and practise hinging at the hips. You will drop the shoulder and reach more on the one hand clean to stretch the lat and better load the contralateral glute to generate more force.
- Gripping the bell too tightly. Keep enough of a grip on the bell so that it doesn't slip out of your hands, but it should be able to move freely within the fingers.
- Rack too far across the chest (see figure 9.13). Many individuals hold the kettlebell too far across the chest or too central. Hold both hands up in a double rack position, even though only one bell is being held, to ensure the positioning is correct and will not need to be altered when progressing to two kettlebells.

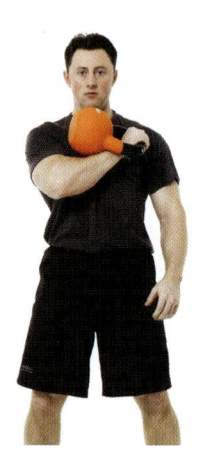

Figure 9.13 Don't have the bell too far across the body in the rack position.

Additional notes
- The load for the one hand clean is about the same weight for the two hand swing.
- Develop good posterior chain strength and endurance prior to using the one hand clean.
- Vary your position slightly to find the optimal placement of hips, knees and bell.
- Master the rack position (exercise 12, page 74) before progressing to the one hand clean.
- Use the rigid style for short sets, with more strength emphasis, and the fluid style for longer sets, with more strength-endurance emphasis.
- Use as an integrated 'lifting-pulling pattern' exercise within your training programme.

Exercise variations
One hand (swing) clean wall drill
The normal swing clean is performed standing close to a wall. This is a great drill to teach the correct bell trajectory. If the kettlebell is swung too far forward and not kept close to the body, then performing the exercise facing a wall helps to solve this. As the kettlebell is lifted, or during the eccentric (lowering) phase, if it travels too far forward it will come into contact with the wall.

ONE HAND FRONT SQUAT

The squat pattern is one of the fundamental human movement patterns. It can be performed with almost any piece of equipment from barbells and dumbbells to cables and powerbags. The parallel stance squat, where both feet are positioned next to each other (exercise 17e and f) is the initial squat pattern to master, prior to a split stance, lunge, or single leg progression.

There is some ambiguity between different organisations about the correct technique to employ for the squat. This includes what depth should be sought, whether the knees should move forward of the toes and the optimal foot positioning. There is an excellent paper published by the National Strength and Conditioning Association (NSCA) in the United States reviewing all the research up to that point on squatting (Chandler & Stone, 1991). This discusses many of the controversial areas that cause debate within the fitness industry. In brief, however, it is recommended to always work through a full range of motion, which includes squatting, as long as there are no restrictions that affect technique or injuries or conditions that may be worsened using a full squat technique. Feet should be positioned in an athletic stance, which can be estimated by adopting the same stance used during a vertical jump, i.e. feet between hip and shoulder width apart. In relation to the knee position, this varies from individual to individual depending on their biomechanics. Focus on keeping the lower leg (shin) and the upper torso parallel, rather than whether the knees do or do not move beyond the toes.

Exercise 17 One hand front squat

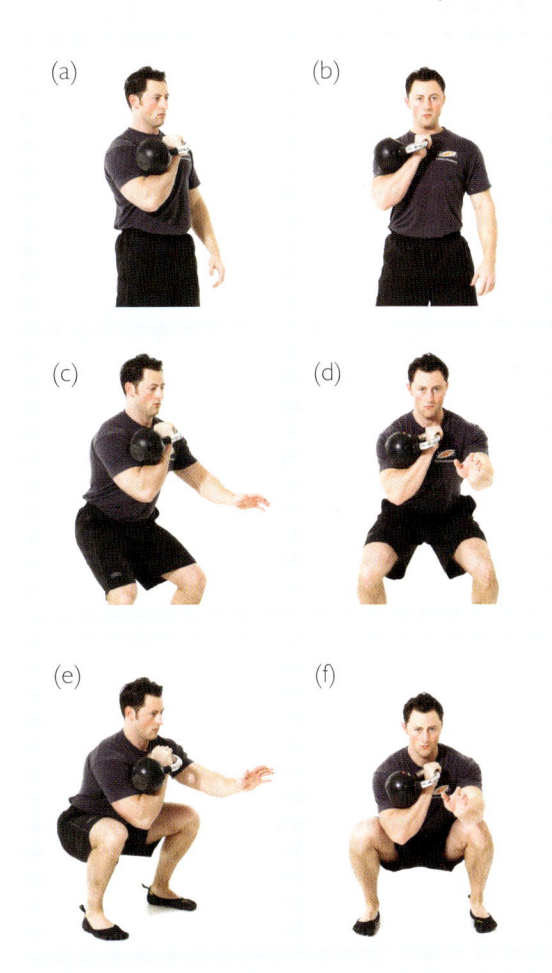

(a) (b)
(c) (d)
(e) (f)

Aims

The aims of the one hand front squat are to teach a squat pattern technique and to work the posterior chain and knee extensor muscles in a squat pattern.

Set-up

- Position the body with feet about hip to shoulder width apart and the kettlebell held in one hand in the rack position.

- The chest should be high with the spine in a neutral position.

Execution
- Brace the core to stabilise and protect the back.
- Push the knees forward and drop into a deep squat using the hip flexors to 'pull' you into position. Keep the torso as vertical as possible.
- Squat down until the distal hamstrings touch the proximal calves, or until technique falters. Ensure the knees and toes are in alignment (patella tracking over the second or third toe) throughout the descent.
- Hold the position for 1–3 seconds without losing tension or relaxing.
- From the deep squat position push the hips forward and drive out of the position, releasing the air from the lungs during the ascent.
- Extend the knees and hips to return to the standing start position and repeat

Key points
- Use the hip flexors to 'pull' you into position.
- Push the hips forward to start the concentric phase.
- Keep feet flat and knees aligned over toes throughout both the descent and ascent.

Key errors
- Heels lifting up (see figure 9.14). This is generally due to poor foot mobility, limited ankle dorsiflexion or having the weight (kettlebell) positioned too far forward.
- Knees caving in (see figure 9.15). This is typical of an overpronation pattern, indicative of weak abductors, tight adductors or a weak vastus medialis obliquus (VMO). Knees should track over the second or third toe.
- Rounding of the back (see figure 9.16). This may be due to limited foot or ankle mobility, so the degree of dorsiflexion should be assessed. If this is the case, then the rounding is occurring to maintain balance. Premature or excessive posterior tilting of the pelvis also causes the back to round. This is usually due to restrictions or poor mobility at the hip.
- Not going to full depth. Limitations at the foot, ankle or hips decrease the individual's ability to squat down to full depth. Always remember you should try to work through a full range of motion with an exercise.
- Keeping knees back/leaning too far forward. Commonly taught as the correct way to squat, this loads the spine more and decreases mobility in the ankles. You should have a similar angle between the lower leg and the torso when squatting down.

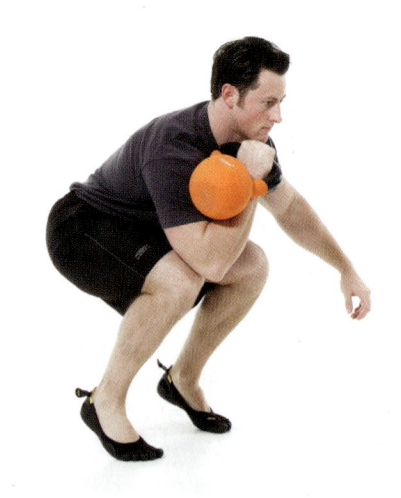

Figure 9.14 Avoid lifting the heels.

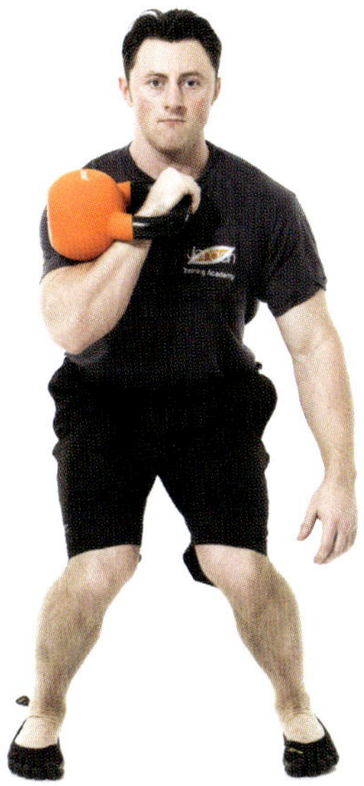

Figure 9.15 Aim to keep knees tracked over the second or third toe.

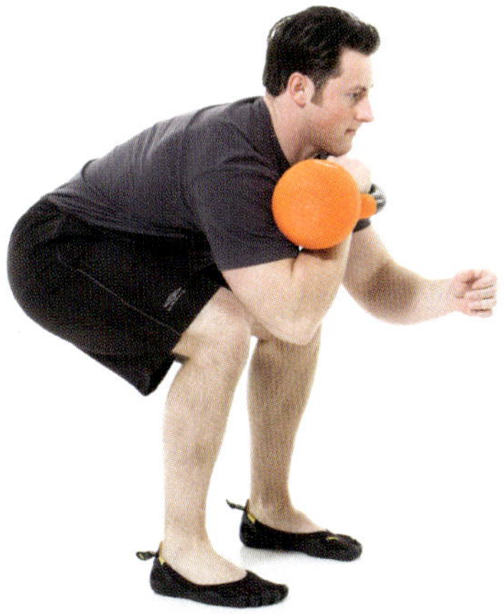

Figure 9.16 Rounding the back can be due to poor ankle mobility.

Additional notes
- Develop good mobility with bodyweight full squats.
- Master the rack position (exercise 12, page 74) before progressing to the one hand front squat.
- Use as a 'squat pattern' exercise within your training programme.

Exercise variations
Front squat heels elevated with one kettlebell
For those that struggle to achieve a full range of motion in the one hand squat, performing the exercise with heels raised can be a useful alternative. If limited ankle or foot mobility decreases the required dorsiflexion, then it is common to see the upper torso leaning forward and/or rounding over to maintain the centre of mass over the base of support. If this didn't happen, the individual would simply fall backwards. If raising the heels on a mat, weight plates or even the handles of two kettlebells laid flat on the ground allows for a full range of motion (full knee flexion) with good shin-to-back positioning, then it should be advocated. This teaches the body to go to a full depth, can help to mobilise the foot and ankle, and helps to strengthen the knee stabilisers, particularly the VMO. This should be accompanied with additional foot, ankle and calf mobilisation, stretching or myofascial release techniques.

Do not rely on having the heels raised to be able to do a full squat; try to achieve this with the feet flat on the ground within 10–12 weeks. Even if the individual does have optimal range of motion, and can perform full squats with the feet flat, this drill can provide a useful variation to be implemented at certain points during the training cycle to alter the stimulus and continue to provide adaptations.

ONE HAND OVERHEAD PRESS

The standing overhead press is one of the most fundamental movements in weightlifting, both modern and ancient. The test of a man's strength always used to be what weight he could lift above his head rather than what he could lift when lying on his back, which seems to be the modern gold standard test (i.e. the bench press).

The standing overhead press requires adequate mobility at the hips, thoracic spine and shoulder rotators, as well as hip, core and shoulder stability. It forms part of the press human movement pattern (a vertical upwards press), alongside pressing horizontally and pressing vertically downwards. This 'strict' press technique minimises involvement of the legs (such as in a push press), momentum (such as in the jerk), or other potential muscle involvement (such as during the side press or bent press).

Exercise 18 One hand overhead press

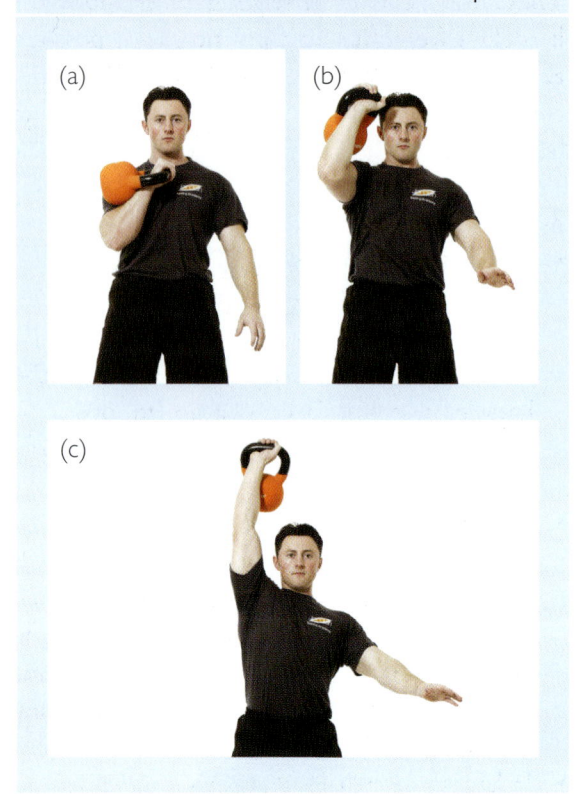

(a) (b) (c)

Aims

The aims of the one hand overhead press exercise are to teach an overhead press technique and to work the pressing muscles and lateral core stabilisers.

Set-up

- Begin in a standing position, feet hip-shoulder width apart.
- Hold the kettlebell in one hand in the rack position.

Execution

There are a couple of techniques to move the kettlebell from the rack position to a position above the head with the arm locked. Brace the core to stabilise and protect the back to initiate both methods.

Method one

- Press the kettlebell straight upwards, rotating the arm during the movement to finish with the palm facing forwards.
- Hold at the top with the arm locked and the handle, not the bell, positioned over the shoulder and hip. The bell should sit slightly behind the body.
- Lower back to the start position and repeat.
- This is the same trajectory used during the push press and jerk, and is similar to the dumbbell Arnold press (which involves starting with one or two dumbbells held on the chest with palms facing the body, and pressing overhead while rotating the palms to face away).
- It keeps the bell closer to the mid-line and requires slightly less lateral stability of the core, but is challenging on the anterior deltoid and thoracic mobility.

Method two

- The second method, preferred by many trainers, is to lift the elbow up and out as if performing a lateral raise.
- Continue the movement by pressing the kettlebell into a full lock position and hold.
- Lower the kettlebell by actively pulling the bell into the body using the latissimus dorsi, until it settles back into the rack position. Hold briefly, then repeat.
- This technique takes the bell slightly further from the midline and thus requires more lateral core and hip stability.
- It can help to develop strength for the pressing muscles in a very strict technique, which can later be applied into a side press.

Key points

- Brace the core and hips to maintain a solid base.
- For this strict variation of the press exercise limit any lateral hip movement and avoid stabilising the hips with the other hand.
- Pull the kettlebell into the body during the eccentric phase

Key errors

- Not keeping the core braced. This results in compensatory movements as you try to press and power leakages. Imagine you are keeping your body rigid while pressing yourself underneath the kettlebell. A common compensation pattern is an anterior pelvic tilt (see figure 9.17), with an increase in the curvature of the lower back. If an individual complains of feeling excessive tension or pain in the lower back when pressing overhead, look at the position of the pelvis, the curvature in the lumbar spine and whether the core is sufficiently activated.
- Not reaching full lockout. It is commonly taught that locking the joints is bad. When using heavy loads it is essential to lockout (not hyperextend) the elbow. Always remember you should try to work through a full range of motion with an exercise.
- Cocked wrist at the top position (see figure 9.18). The wrist should be rigid and straight throughout the full duration of the exercise, from the rack to the press position.

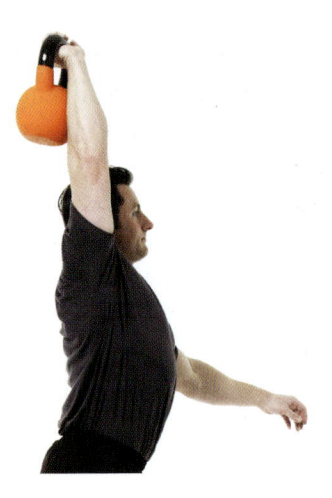

Figure 9.17 Anterior pelvic tilt can result in lower back pain.

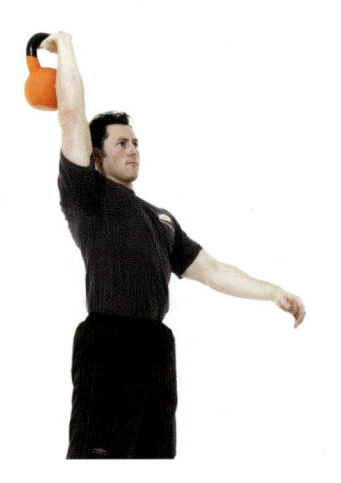

Figure 9.18 Do not cock the wrist at the top position.

- The kettlebell is too far forward at the locked press position (see figure 9.19). This is usually due to restrictions in the thoracic spine or medial rotators of the shoulder.

- The kettlebell is too far out to the side (see figure 9.20). Some individuals struggle to raise their arm straight above their head because of shoulder or thoracic restrictions and may finish the exercise too far out to the side. The bell should be over the hip and shoulder, looking from the front or the side.

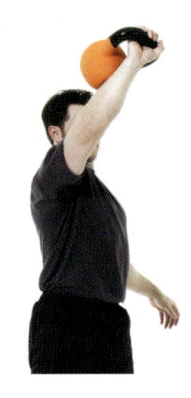

Figure 9.19 Do not let the kettlebell move too far forward.

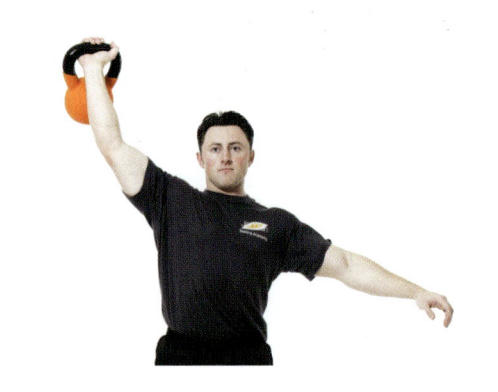

Figure 9.20 The bell should be over the hip and shoulder with a straight arm.

Additional notes

- Master the rack position (exercise 12, page 74) before progressing to the one hand overhead press.
- Use as part of the 'press or push pattern' within your training programme.
- The door drill can be used to teach a rigid body position; stand under a doorframe and try to push it upwards. This teaches the core and hips to not 'give in' against a heavy load.

ONE HAND TURKISH GET-UP

The Turkish get-up is a rarely seen drill in many of today's gyms and health clubs, yet a hundred years ago it was a staple exercise in a weightlifter's programme. This variation involves moving a kettlebell from a supine position on the floor to an overhead standing position and is grouped as a 'moving' or 'carrying load' human movement pattern.

The Turkish get-up can also be performed using a dumbbell, barbell, fitbar or powerbag for different benefits. It requires mobility and stability in the shoulder and shoulder girdle, core stability, hip mobility and concentration.

There are no specific prerequisite exercises to perform the Turkish get-up, apart from ensuring optimal thoracic, shoulder and hip mobility with stretches and self-myofascial release. When learning the exercise, however, it can be split into five different phases, which can be taught separately and then integrated together:

- Phase 1: Supine to upright seated position
- Phase 2: Hip and leg lift
- Phase 3: Leg sweep underneath
- Phase 4: Split kneeling position
- Phase 5: Split kneeling to standing

Exercise 19 One hand Turkish get-up from supine with one kettlebell

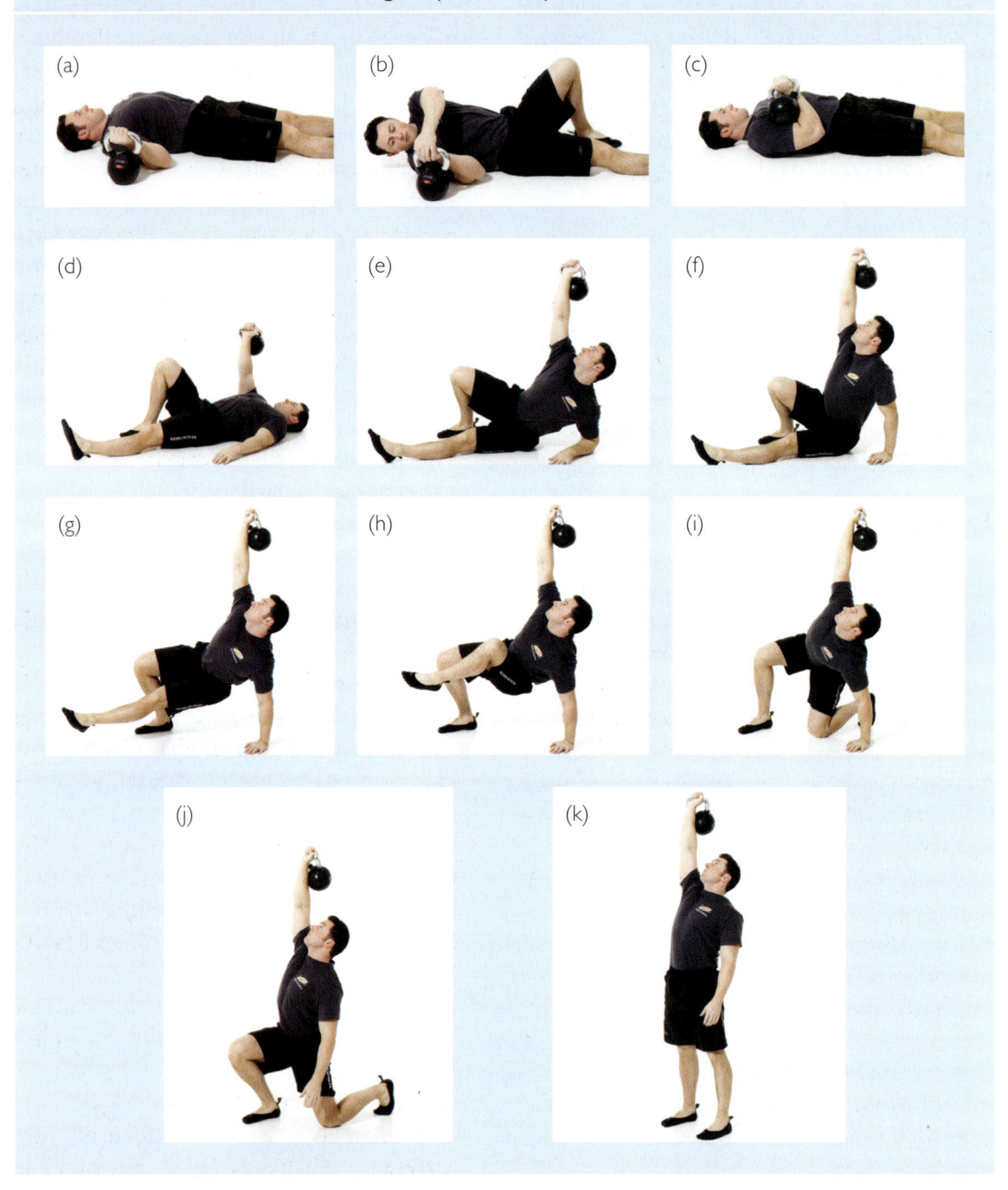

Aims

The aims of the Turkish get-up are to teach the body to move under load from a supine to a standing position; to mobilise and strengthen the shoulder and shoulder girdle muscles; and to develop strength in the stabilising muscles of the anterior and lateral core.

Set-up

- Lie in a supine position (facing the ceiling) with the kettlebell side on next to one shoulder.
- Roll towards the kettlebell and grip the handle with both hands (exercise 19).
- Pull the kettlebell on to the nearest side of the chest/shoulder and roll back into the supine position.

Execution

- Inhale and brace the abdominal wall. Press the kettlebell from the chest into a locked arm position pointing straight upwards. Focus on keeping the arm in a straight vertical position throughout the different phases. Watch the kettlebell at all times throughout both the concentric and eccentric phases.
- The contralateral (opposite side) arm should be extended on the floor at about 45 degrees from the body. Bend the knee of the ipsilateral (same side) leg and place the foot flat on the ground.
- Push the kettlebell upwards by lifting the torso from the floor and pushing up on to the contralateral elbow. Then push the body up on to the hand so that the arm is straight and the torso is in a fully upright, seated position.
- Push down with the supporting hand and foot to lift the hips upwards off the floor.
- Bring the knee back to the chest and underneath the body until in a supported kneeling lunge position.
- Lift the supporting hand off the floor using the lateral core until in an unsupported kneeling lunge position. Stand upright so that the feet are parallel, shoulder width apart, with the 'working' arm extended upwards in a locked position.
- To return to the start position, step backwards with the opposite leg, place the hand on the floor, sweep the leg through, hips and extended leg on the floor, lower on to the elbow then lower the shoulders.

Key points

- Watch the kettlebell throughout.
- Undertake each phase slowly.
- Keep the arm extended upwards throughout.

Key errors

- Not keeping the core braced. This results in compensatory movements as you try to get up as the power leaks from the body.
- Not having sufficient space between the hips and the supporting hand. This makes it very difficult to 'sweep' the leg through when the hips are lifted up.
- Not looking at the kettlebell throughout. This usually allows the arm to bend or move from an upright position, causing the kettlebell to fall or balance to be lost. Ensure eyes are fixed on the kettlebell throughout.
- Arm not locked. Ensure the elbow of the 'working' arm is locked at all times to prevent any collapses.
- Overextending the hips (see figure 9.21 overleaf). This is used to try to mobilise the anterior hip (hip flexors) but can stress some of the structures of the back.

Additional notes
- Break down the phases into different sections when learning.
- Keep the reps low as the time-under-tension (TUT) for each rep is quite long.
- Use as a moving-carrying exercise within your training programme to improve core and shoulder stability.

ONE HAND WINDMILL

The windmill is a fantastic exercise for improving lateral core strength and for shoulder stability and mobility. Unlike the swing, clean and snatch, the windmill is more of a low tempo, high isometric stabilisation exercise.

Many people look at the windmill and question its carryover to basic movement patterns like the lift, squat, press or pull. The windmill looks more like a weighted yoga move than an exercise seen in the modern gym or health club. However, it is probably *the* foundation drill for any exercise that requires frontal plane stability. The one hand kettlebell windmill is a strength and stability exercise, categorised as a remedial drill for unilateral pressing or lifting movements. It develops the lateral core, hip stability and shoulder mobility and stability essential when pressing a load above the head in one hand or when lifting a weight from the floor with one hand.

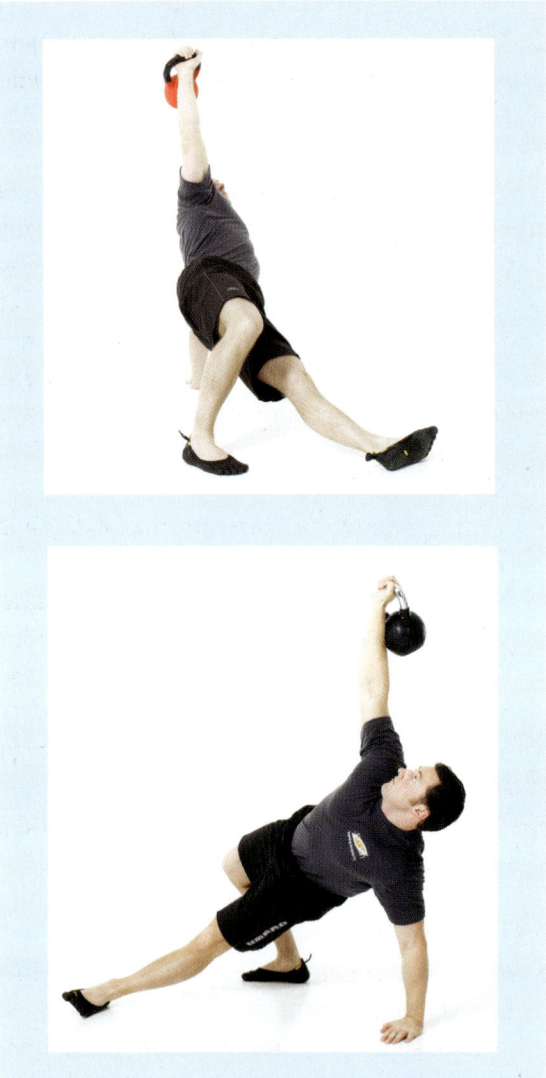

Figure 9.21 Avoid overextending the hips.

Exercise 20 One hand windmill

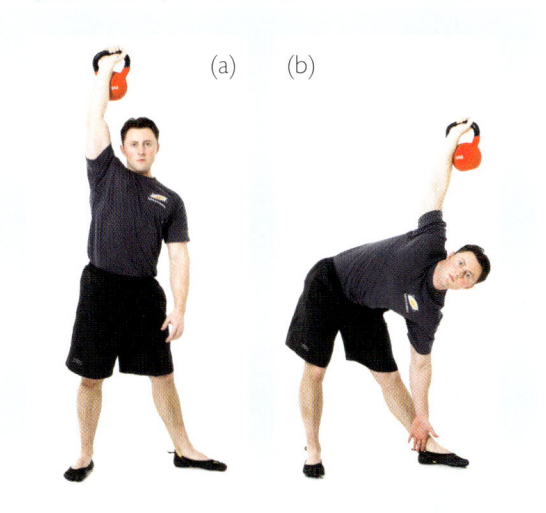

(a)   (b)

Aims
The aims of the one hand windmill are to develop frontal plane stability for unilateral lifting or pressing; to work the lateral core and hip stabilisers; and to develop shoulder mobility and stability for overhead pressing.

Set-up
- Lift the kettlebell up to the overhead press position (exercise 18, page 82), using the clean and press or snatch techniques as previously described.
- Then, with the feet about hip to shoulder width apart, adopt one of the following stance positions depending on what feels most comfortable:
  1. Turn the opposite foot out at about 90 degrees keeping the knee stiff (b).
  2. Turn both feet out about 30 degrees with the heels on the same line, keeping the opposite knee stiff.
  3. Turn both feet out about 30 degrees again, but allowing the opposite knee to bend slightly.

The third option works best for many because of the lack of hamstring range of motion many individuals present with. Marc (pictured) has excellent lower body flexibility and thus feels most comfortable with the knee stiff. Turn the opposite arm so that the back of the hand is against the inner thigh of the 'leading' leg.

Execution
- Inhale and brace the core, creating abdominal pressure.
- Many people like to look though the kettlebell to a point on the ceiling throughout this drill.
- Push the rear hip (the one beneath the kettlebell) over the rear foot.
- Slide the back of the hand down the inner thigh and lower leg.
- Pause briefly at the bottom, then return to the start position to repeat the process.

Key points
- Watch the kettlebell throughout the drill when held above the head.
- Undertake each rep slowly, taking 3–4 seconds on the way down with a 1–2 second hold at the bottom.
- Keep the arm extended vertically upwards throughout the drill.
- Push the hip out and over the rear foot.

Key errors
- Weight shifting over the front leg (see figure 9.22). When the hips move towards the lead leg, it takes the tension off the hip stabilisers

FOUNDATION EXERCISES

and puts more stress on the lateral core. These muscles should work together to stabilise the hips and core during this drill. To correct this, have the individual perform the exercise with the rear hip touching a wall so that they can feel when it moves off.

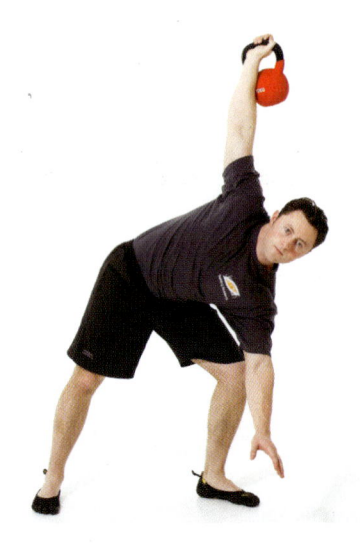

Figure 9.22 Don't allow the hips to move towards the lead leg.

Exercise 21 One hand windmill with hands behind the back

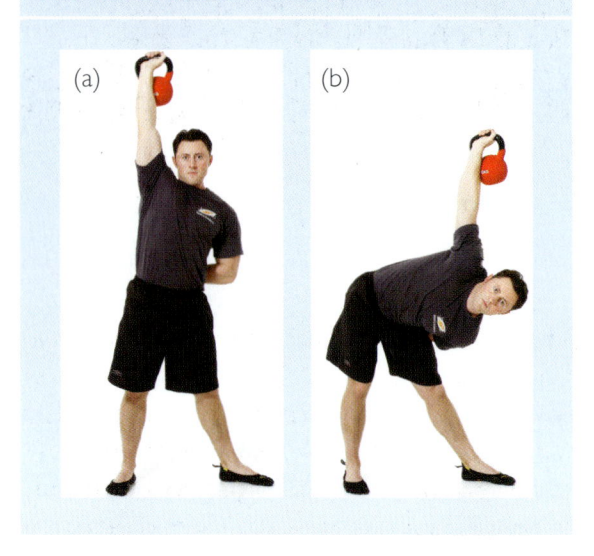

(a) (b)

Execution
- Place the other hand behind the back as if scratching an itch between the shoulder blades. This allows for a greater range of motion and further challenges the working muscles.

Exercise variations

The following progressions can be applied to the windmill exercise:

- One hand windmill with one kettlebell held in lower hand
- One hand windmill with one kettlebell held in upper hand
- One hand windmill with one kettlebell held in upper hand with lower hand held behind the back (see exercise 21)
- Two hand windmill with two kettlebells, one held in each hand.

EXERCISE PROGRESSIONS 10

These progressions allow you to add variety to training sessions, while still overloading many of the same muscles or chains of muscles. The variations overload the body in a slightly different way, which allows you to adapt your programme for your specific requirements. You may find some drills easier and more preferable, but it is always good to try a variety of these to achieve balance within the body.

Most of these are described as 'progressions' and, as such, should only be performed when the original drill has been carried out and the technique mastered.

SWING VARIATIONS

Exercise 22 Two hand rack Girevoy style

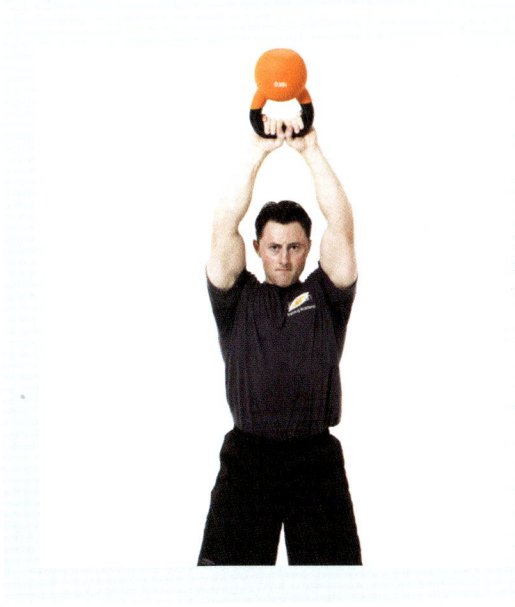

Also known as an American swing, this is a variation of the standard (Russian) two hand swing, but the finish point is with the kettlebell in a much higher position overhead, which requires more deceleration of the anterior chain abdominal muscles.

Set-up
- Start as you do for the two hand swing with a parallel stance and the feet approximately shoulder width apart.
- Position the kettlebell with the handle aligned between the heels.
- Bend forwards from the hips, keeping a neutral spine.
- Aim the hips back to activate the hamstrings and glutes.

Execution
- Take a breath in, hold it and brace the core muscles.
- Contract the muscles of the glutes and hamstrings to quickly bring the hips forward to a fully extended (upright) position with as much controlled force as you can. This movement should drive the kettlebell upwards (you are aiming for an overhead position with the kettlebell finishing upside down, right above the head but just slightly forward of vertical).
- As you reach the maximal height with the kettlebell, strongly contract the abdominal muscles to decelerate the motion of the bell and stabilise in a standing position at the top.
- As the kettlebell drops, guide it back towards the groin and between the legs, hinging the hips back as you would with the traditional (Russian) swing and repeat.

Exercise variations
There is another variation of this drill, called the crescent swing, where the bell is lifted completely over the head and the body turns on a point 180 degrees to allow the bell to swing through the legs, but facing the opposite way. Although some like this variation it is quite probable that the kettlebell will hit the shins at some point, causing injury. Any benefit that may be gained from this variation is outweighed by the risk of injury.

Exercise 23 Two hand swing with two kettlebells

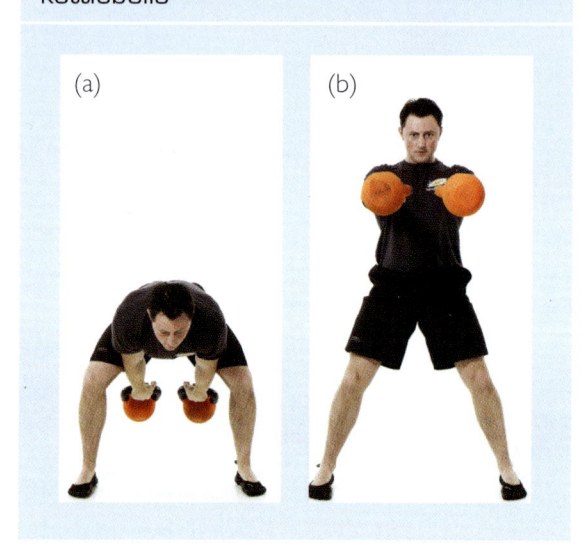

This is a similar drill to the two hand swing (Exercise 5, page 57), but you use two separate kettlebells, one held in each hand. This requires more coordination and should only be undertaken when the two hand and one hand swings have been mastered. The set-up is the same postural position as with the two hand swing with one kettlebell, but usually with the legs slightly wider.

Execution
- Start with one kettlebell in each hand in between the legs, and then drive the hips forwards to project the two kettlebells forwards and upwards.

- Keep the hands pronated (palms facing down) throughout.
- Use a much lighter weight when first attempting this drill, and progress gradually.

Exercise 24 Two hand swing with lateral step, with one kettlebell

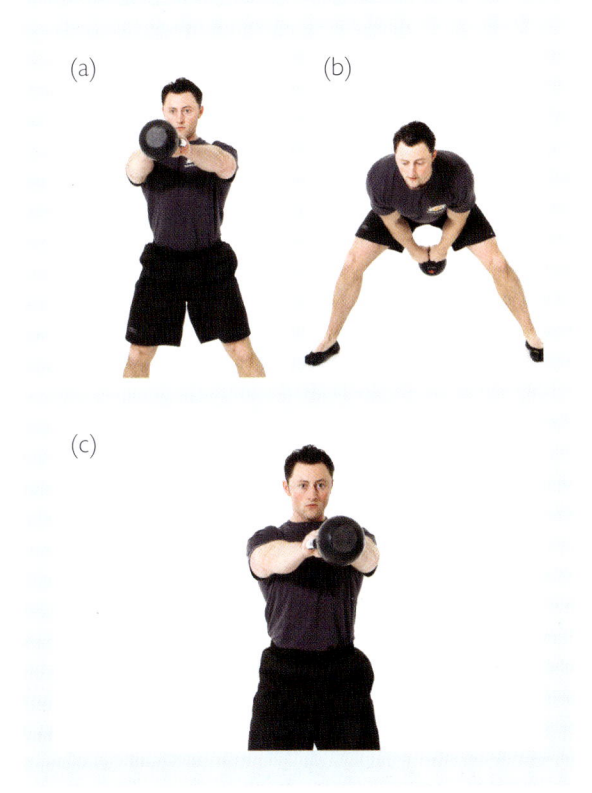

(a)   (b)

(c)

This variation of the swing adds an additional dimension to the challenge on the body. It recruits the core stabilisers and moves the body through the frontal plane, which is often ignored in a standard training programme. Including frontal plane movements helps to balance the workouts, which can be dominated by Sagittal plane exercises.

Execution
- With this drill, perform the kettlebell swing as normal, then as the bell reaches shoulder height and becomes weightless, and it begins to fall, take a lateral step: this wide stance is adopted to prepare for the bell to return between the legs.
- Allow the kettlebell to swing in between the thighs, and then as the kettlebell swings upwards bring the legs together again.
- Repeat for several reps, alternating direction with each rep to ensure that the right and left hand sides of the body are worked equally.

Exercise variations
Other swing variations involving movement include:

- Two hand swing walking forwards
- Two hand swing walking backwards
- Two hand swing walking laterally

Exercise 25 Two hand swing with one kettlebell and towel/rope

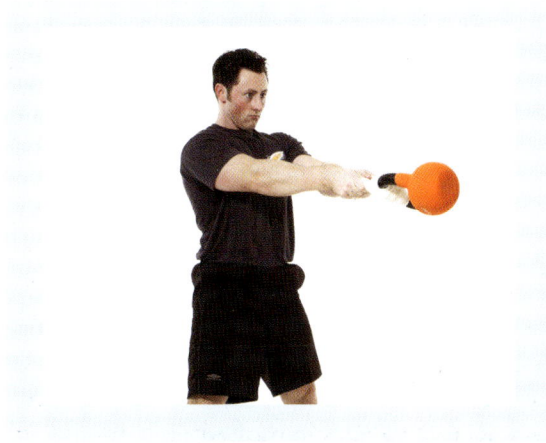

This is essentially the two hand swing (exercise 5, page 57), but using a towel increases the lever length, which helps to increase the overload on the posterior chain muscles. It also provides a grip challenge to the muscles of the hand and forearm.

Execution
- To perform this drill, thread a towel through the handle of the kettlebell and hold the towel with both hands, trying to position the bell centrally on the towel.
- Execute the two hand swing.
- A safety point to consider: Ensure that the towel is not too long and that you can perform the swing pattern without hitting the floor. Using a hand towel rather than a bath towel is recommended. It may also work better to stand on two steps so that the kettlebell can swing between them without hitting the floor.

Exercise 26 Two hand swing partner-added push (power bomb) with one kettlebell

This exercise variation requires a partner who is knowledgeable about kettlebell training.

Execution
- The partner stands in front, outside of the swing arc, and facing forwards.
- As the individual swings the bell and it reaches the peak of its arc at chest/shoulder height, the partner should place their hands on the top of the bell and 'throw' it downwards as it starts to drop. This additional force causes the bell to accelerate quicker between the legs and causes a greater loading effect on the posterior chain muscles.
- Allow the bell to go between the thighs as normal and accelerate the bell upwards using a powerful hip extension to repeat the process.
- Gradually build up the force exerted on the bell and always ensure the partner is far enough outside the natural arc so as not to get hit.

Exercise 27 Hand-to-hand swing with one kettlebell

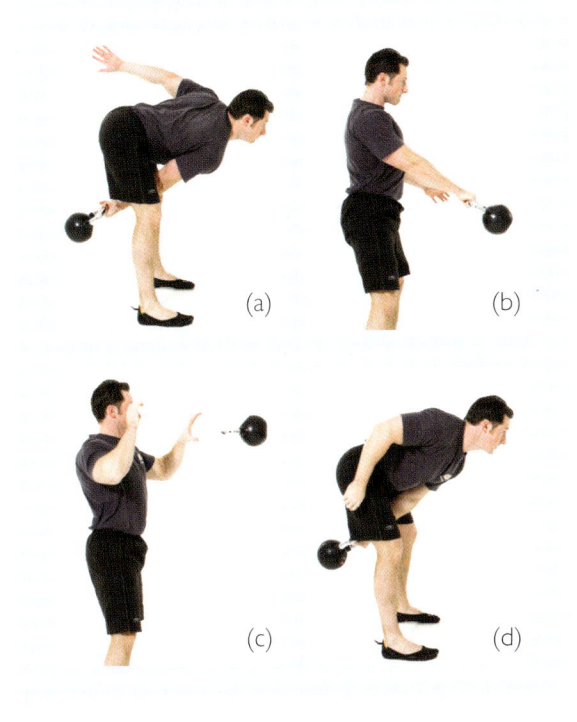

(a) (b) (c) (d)

This is a variation of the one hand swing (exercise 9, page 65), which is good preparation for the more advanced juggling drills described later in the book. This drill alternates the load of the core and leg muscles from left to right, challenges the grip and proprioception and gets the individual used to releasing the bell and not lifting with the upper body.

Execution
- Start the one hand swing as normal with the feet hip width apart and the bell between the legs in preparation for a swing action. It is easier to perform this variation with a rotated palm; with the thumb leading the hand holding the kettlebell as it swings between the legs.
- As the bell is swung forwards, rotate the arm so that the palm faces downwards (pronated) and release at this moment to catch with the opposite hand.
- Then, finish the second phase of the swing with this arm, rotating the palm so that the thumb is facing backwards at the end of the movement.
- As this is repeated, there is naturally an alternation between the right and left on the different phases of the swing cycle.

Exercise variations
If this seems a little too challenging then swing the kettlebell with one hand finishing in a semi-supinated position with the palm facing inwards. As the kettlebell reaches the peak of the swing, take hold of the handle with both hands (one either side) then release the first hand and swap other. This is the most basic of the hand-to-hand swings, since the kettlebell is never fully released.

Exercise 28 One hand swing with one kettlebell and release at the top

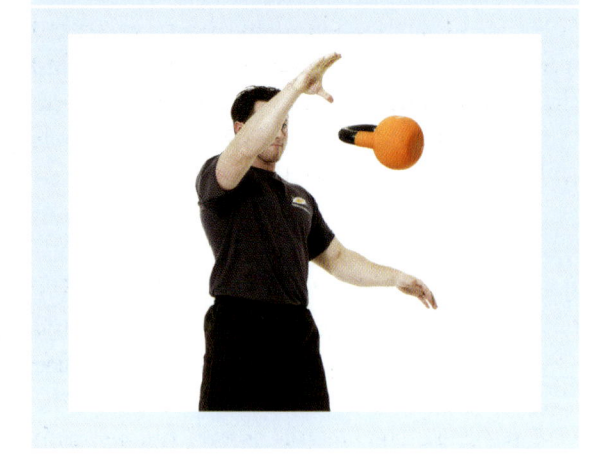

The benefits of releasing the bell in this drill are greater hand-eye coordination and an increased eccentric loading phase as the bell is re-caught and the body has to stabilise this dynamic load before it falls to the floor. This drill can also increase the quality of detail in all one hand swings, as when the kettlebell is released there should be no extraneous movement of the bell. At the point of release it should stay still, without flipping or twisting. The less movement of the bell, the more efficient and fluid the swing technique must be.

Execution
- As with the standard one hand swing, the set-up and starting swing phase are the same. The difference comes at the end range of the movement, as the bell reaches its maximal height.
- As the bell starts to become weightless at the point of transition, momentarily release it before re-catching it as it begins to fall.
- Finish the drill by guiding the bell between the legs at the bottom of the movement as you would with any swing.

Exercise 29 One hand swing with one kettlebell and fingers release

A regression of the actual release, this is a great drill for building up the confidence to completely let go of the handle.

Execution
- Proceed as you would for exercise 28.
- As the kettlebell swings up release the grip of the fingers, but keep part of the palm in contact with the handle.
- Re-grip as the bell starts to drop and repeat.

Exercise 30 One hand swing with one kettlebell and Sagittal flip

In this drill the kettlebell is not only released, but is deliberately flipped in the Sagittal plane (upwards and backward through 360 degrees), as if the bell is doing a somersault.

Execution
- Proceed as you would for exercise 28.
- When the bell is weightless, flip the handle underneath and around.
- After the handle has rotated around the bell, grip it with the same hand, swing it in between the legs and repeat.

Exercise 31 One hand swing with one kettlebell and frontal flip

To picture how to carry out this drill, hold your arm out straight in front of you at shoulder height. Start with the thumb pointing down and rotate until the thumb is pointing up. In this horizontal position, this would be the same rotation occurring with the kettlebell.

Execution
- Proceed as you would for exercise 28 (page 96), but start with the thumb facing backwards, and the palm rotated outwards.
- As the bell is swung forwards, release it and simultaneously rotate the hand so that the thumb faces upwards and the palm inwards.
- As the handle of the bell rotates around keep the hand in the same position, with the thumb pointing down, and catch the bell in this position.
- Swing the bell between the legs as usual and repeat.

Exercise 32 One hand swing with one kettlebell and transverse flip

In this variation, the kettlebell is rotated transversely, as if the handle is travelling around the equator. The other way of explaining it is to imagine the kettlebell is a turntable and the handle rotates around the bell as if in a flat spin.

Execution
- Proceed as you would for exercise 28 (page 96).
- As the bell is swung forwards, release it and simultaneously spin the handle to the outside and away.
- The handle should spin around the bell as it hangs in mid-air, as if moving around the 'equator of the bell'.
- As the handle spins back round catch it, swing the bell between the legs as usual and repeat.

Exercise 33 One hand swing with two kettlebells

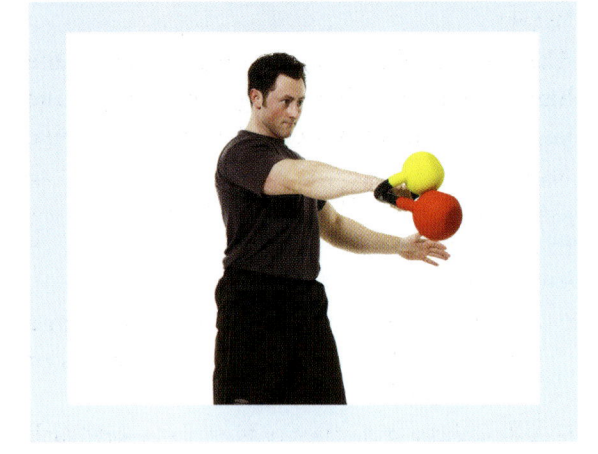

Exercise 34 One hand swing with one kettlebell and a towel

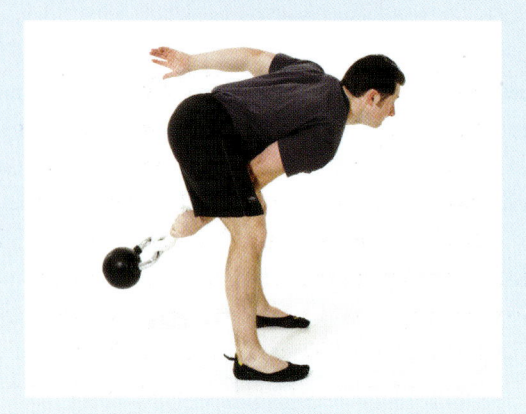

This drill will massively increase the load on the muscles of the forearm and is an ideal exercise for those looking to increase their grip strength.

Execution
- Using two kettlebells, hold both handles in one hand, by drawing the handles to meet as close as possible.
- The bells need to be held tightly throughout to avoid any lateral swinging of the weights as you perform the usual swing action.

This is a one hand variation of the two hand swing with a towel (exercise 25, page 93) and is great for improving grip strength and endurance.

Execution
- Thread a towel through the handle of the kettlebell and hold the towel with one hand, trying to position the bell centrally on the towel.
- Execute the one hand swing.
- A safety point to consider: ensure that the towel is not too long and that you can perform the swing pattern without hitting the floor. Using a hand towel rather than a bath towel is recommended. It may also work better to stand on two steps so that the kettlebell can swing between them without hitting the floor.

Exercise variations
Other one hand swing variations include:

- One hand swing and lateral step (or swing with side step)

- One hand swing walking forwards
- One hand swing walking backwards
- One hand swing walking laterally

DEADLIFT EXERCISES

The lift pattern is probably the most utilised of all the movement patterns within kettlebell training. The two hand swing, one hand swing, clean and snatch all incorporate the lift patterning of hip flexion and extension with core and back stabilisation, whether it makes up the entire movement for that particular exercise or it is a part of the drill.

There are many other lifting exercises from the dead position that can be performed with one or more kettlebells. Most of these can form essential progressions to improve strength, endurance or stability, which will have a positive carryover to the more ballistic lift pattern kettlebell exercises, such as the swing, snatch and clean.

Exercise 35 Good morning one kettlebell on the back

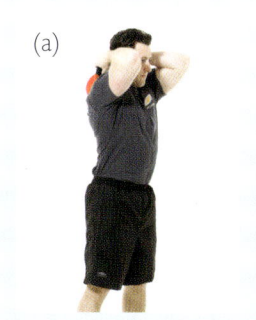

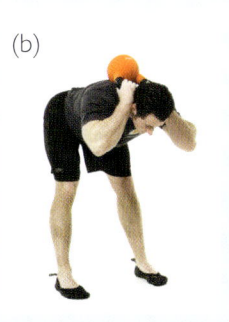

(a)   (b)

This position requires a certain amount of shoulder rotation and may not be comfortable for everyone. There are plenty of alternative exercises to overload the posterior chain muscles if this is the case, such as any of the deadlifts or swings.

Aims

The aims of this exercise are to mobilise the lumbar spine and hamstrings; to overload the posterior chain of muscles (hamstrings, calves, upper and lower back); and to encourage strong posture in the upper back and shoulders.

Set-up
- Start with the feet about hip width apart in a parallel standing position, facing forwards or with a slight external rotation.
- Either have a partner pass you the kettlebell from behind, or carefully lift the weight overhead to rest on the fleshy part of the upper back, holding it by the handle in both hands with the palms facing inwards, towards the head, elbows pointing outwards.

Execution
- The chest should be high with the spine in a neutral position (slight curvature in the low back) or flat, but definitely not rounded. The shins should be vertical throughout.
- Take a small breath in and activate (brace) the core, then pull the hips backwards, with a slight bend in both knees, and lower the upper torso towards the floor. Try to get to horizontal (90 degrees of hip flexion) with the chest at least at 45 degrees, depending on lower back and hamstring flexibility.
- Maintain the tension throughout the body as you push the hips forwards to a standing position with the head and chest in neutral. You will need to ensure that the head remains in line with the spine throughout this drill because of the position of the kettlebell.

Exercise 36 Two hand Romanian deadlift (RDL) with one kettlebell

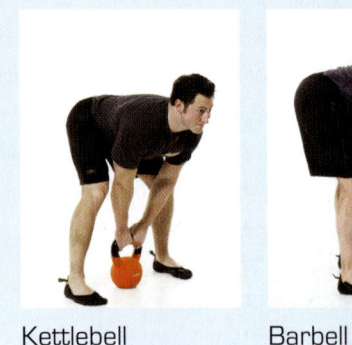

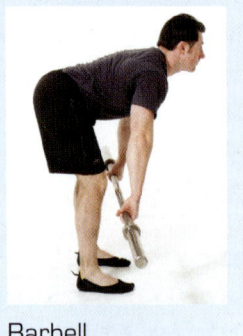

Kettlebell

Barbell

The RDL was described in chapter 7 (figure 7.10, page 39). It is one of the essential lifts to master, demonstrating that a neutral or flat back can be maintained while the hip is flexing on load (holding a weight). It doesn't really matter whether that load is a barbell, dumbbell, kettlebell or other weight. The heaviest loads will always be used with a barbell, but using a kettlebell can help an individual to achieve the correct grip, stance and bell position for many of the kettlebell progression exercises, so it is worth undertaking.

The stiff leg deadlift is a variation on the RDL. The main difference between these exercises is the degree of knee flexion, or exactly how much bending occurs. With a stiff leg deadlift the knees are stiff, but not locked, and move backwards from vertical as the hips move back. This increases the tension of the portion of the hamstrings at the insertion point (where the muscle attaches) near the knees. However, when performing an RDL, the knees remain still and the shins vertical, which causes more knee flexion (about 30 degrees) as the hips move back. This slight knee bend, caused by keeping the shins vertical rather than by squatting down, creates more hamstring tension towards the middle or belly of the hamstrings.

Exercise variations

Some of the variations of these drills include:

- RDL with one kettlebell held with two hands
- RDL with one kettlebell held with one hand
- RDL with two kettlebells held with two hands
- RDL with one kettlebell held with a farmer's hold grip – also referred to as a suitcase deadlift
- RDL with one kettlebell held with crush grip (for grip, see figure 6.8, page 28)
- Stiff leg deadlift with one kettlebell held with two hands
- Stiff leg deadlift with one kettlebell held with one hand
- Stiff leg deadlift with two kettlebells held with two hands
- Stiff leg deadlift with one kettlebell held with two hands
- Stiff leg deadlift with one kettlebell held with a suitcase grip
- Stiff leg deadlift with one kettlebell held with a crush grip
- Stiff leg deadlift with one kettlebell stood on a step to increase range of motion (ROM)

Exercise 37 Two hand sumo deadlift with one kettlebell

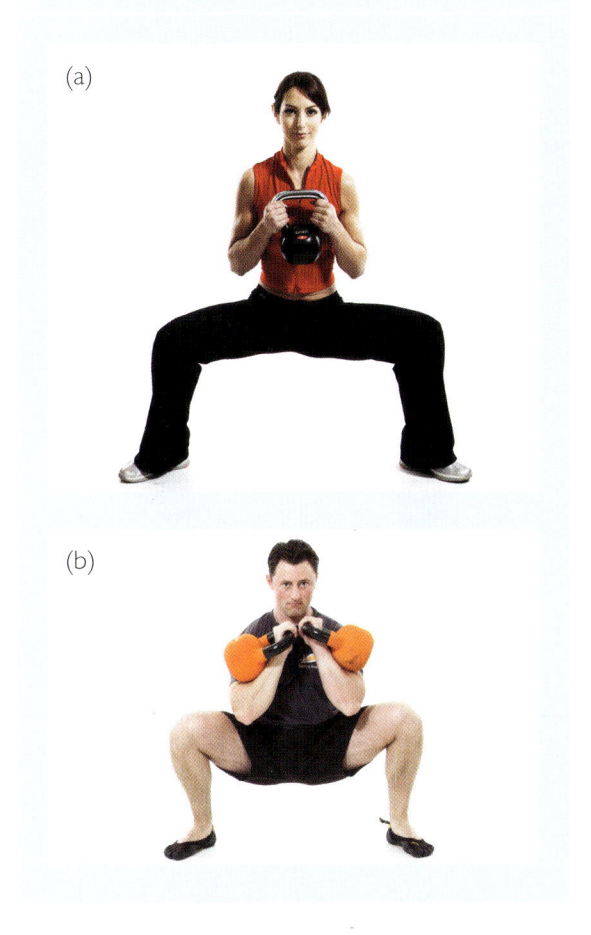

(a)

(b)

The sumo deadlift requires a wide stance, and there is some argument as to whether it can be called a deadlift, since it actually resembles more of a squat pattern. The bell is lifted from the floor with one or both hands, with one or two kettlebells, stood on the floor or elevated up on a step.

The bell can be held on the chest with both hands (a), or in rack (b). It is a sumo deadlift when the bell is lifted from the floor and a sumo squat when the bell is held on the chest or above the head.

Exercise 38 Two hand single leg deadlift with one kettlebell

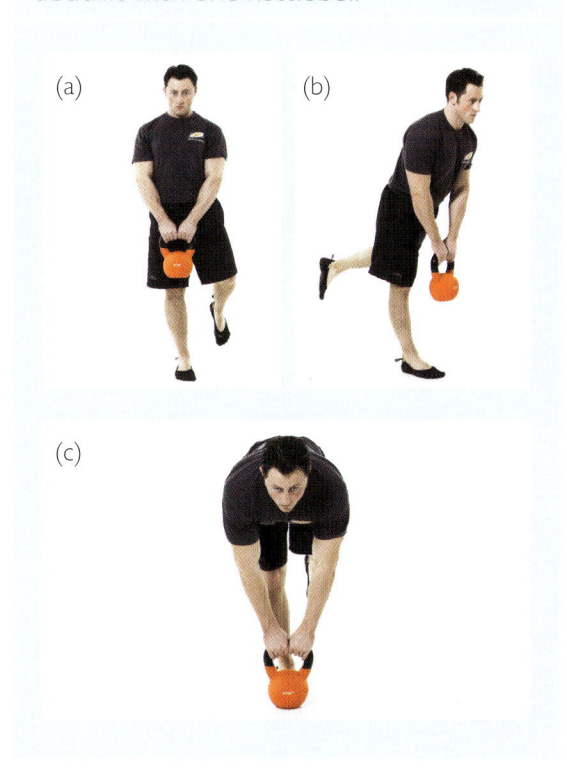

(a) (b)

(c)

This is an excellent drill for improving single leg strength and foot, ankle, knee and hip stability, and it also gets the lateral glutes on the hips firing effectively.

Aims
The aims of this exercise are to teach a single leg lift technique and to work the posterior (extensor) chain muscles in a lifting pattern.

Set-up
- Stand on one foot with the other foot elevated off the floor. Use this other leg for balance throughout the drill.

EXERCISE PROGRESSIONS

101

- Hold the kettlebell with two hands in a normal pronated grip, with the bell held on the lower abdomen or front of the hips.

Execution
- Push the hips back and flex at the hips, while maintaining a correct back position.
- Bend the knee to lower the kettlebell towards the floor and push the foot into the ground, gripping it with the toes.
- Use a hips-knees-knees-hips phase pattern – focus on flexing at the hips first before bending the knees. At the same time extend the other leg behind the body to help maintain balance.
- Touch the bell on the floor, hold briefly and then straighten the knee and extend the hips to lift the kettlebell up.
- Pause at the top and then repeat.

Key errors
- Heels lifting up. This will be due to reaching too far forward with the kettlebell. Keep the kettlebell closer to the body.
- Knees caving in. This is typical of an overpronation pattern, indicative of weak abductors, tight adductors or a weak vastus medialis obliquus (VMO). Knees should track over the second or third toe.
- Rounding of the back. The individual needs to differentiate between hip flexion and spinal flexion, and practice hinging at the hips. This may also be due to a restrictive superficial back line (calves, hamstrings, erector spinae).
- Not going to full depth. Limitations at the hips, such as tight hamstrings, will limit the individual's ability to squat down to full depth.

Exercise variations
Variations of the single leg deadlift include:

- Single leg deadlift with two kettlebells
- Single leg deadlift with one kettlebell and one hand contralateral grip (figure 10.1a)
- Single leg deadlift with one kettlebell and one hand ipsilateral grip (figure 10.1b)
- Single stiff leg deadlift with one kettlebell
- Single stiff leg deadlift with two kettlebells (figure 10.1c)

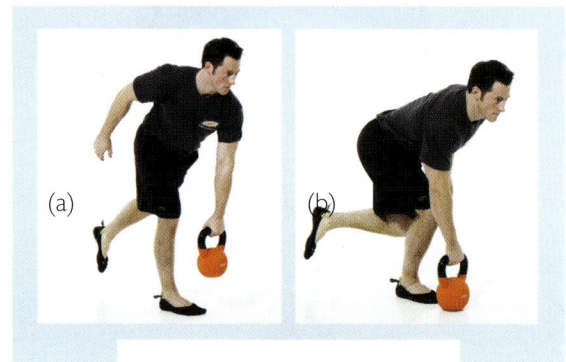

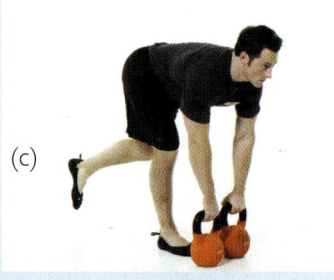

Figure 10.1 Variations of the single leg deadlift: (a) with one kettlebell and a one hand contralateral grip; (b) with one kettlebell and a one hand ipsilateral grip; and (c) with two kettlebells.

SNATCH VARIATIONS

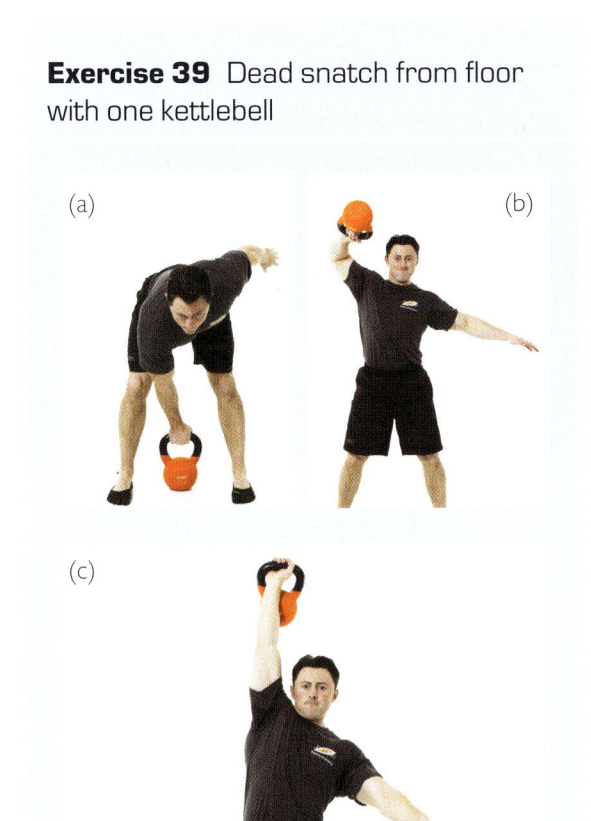

Exercise 39 Dead snatch from floor with one kettlebell

(a)

(b)

(c)

The dead snatch from the floor is a more muscular force development and less elastic, plyometric variation of the standard (swing) snatch. Whereas the standard snatch will have a swing between the legs to load the hamstrings, glutes and lats elastically in order to generate more force and make the concentric load on the muscles easier, the dead snatch does not. There is no preceding eccentric phase, and the muscles must generate the required force to lift the bell above the head without any pre-loading. Because there is no momentum for the previous repetition used, the muscles must generate all of the force themselves. Consequently, more energy is expelled with this variation than with the (swing) snatch. The trajectory of the kettlebell is also more vertical than in the (swing) snatch, and more similar to the barbell variation of this exercise.

Aims

The aims of this exercise are to teach an explosive lifting-pulling technique and to work the posterior (extensor) chain muscles in a lifting pattern.

Set-up

- Begin in deadlift position, feet hip to shoulder width apart with the kettlebell positioned between the heels on the floor.
- Brace the core to stabilise and protect the back.
- Limit knee bend to adequately load the posterior chain.

Execution

- Extend the hips and knees forcibly and aggressively.
- As the kettlebell rises from between the knees, pull forcibly upwards, keeping the kettlebell close to the body.
- Punch upwards to flip the kettlebell handle underneath the bell so that it finishes above the shoulder.
- Pause, then drop the elbow and twist the forearm.
- Guide the kettlebell backwards through the legs to return to the start position and repeat.
- Keep the repetitions low when learning the technique and gradually build up the volume.

EXERCISE PROGRESSIONS

Key points
- Follow a fast 1-2-3 pattern – hips, pull, punch.
- Be very aggressive.
- Pull the bell close to the body.
- Punch quickly upwards with a small range of motion.

Exercise variations
Variations of the dead snatch from the floor include:

- Olympic dead snatch from the floor with one kettlebell. This is the same as exercise 39, but it includes a dip down to catch the kettlebell in an overhead squat position before standing up.
- Dead snatch from the hang position with one kettlebell (exercise 40)
- Dead snatch from the floor stood on a step with one kettlebell
- Dead snatch from the floor with two kettlebells
- Dead snatch from the hang position with two kettlebells
- Diagonal dead snatch from the floor with one kettlebell.

Exercise 40 Hang snatch with one kettlebell

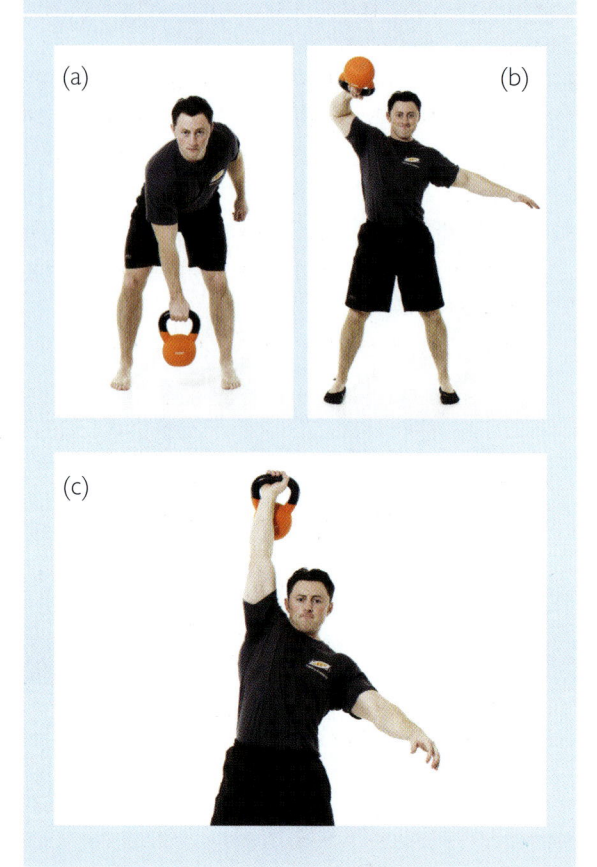

(a) (b) (c)

The hang snatch is a variation of the (swing) snatch where the bell is lifted above the head in one motion, but without the full swing between the legs. The trajectory is more vertical than the arc of the (swing) snatch. Dropping the bell downwards and then immediately changing direction will provide some elastic energy to help lift the bell, but much less than is generated from a full swing between the legs.

Execution
- Start in an upright position, with the bell resting on the front of the hips and the lifting arm straight.
- Bend forward so that the bell drops to about knee or calf height and then immediately change direction by extending the hips and lifting upwards with the arm.
- Punch the kettlebell into the snatch finish position, hold briefly, and then lower to the start position.
- Pause for a second or so and then repeat.

Exercise 41 Dead snatch from the hang position with one kettlebell

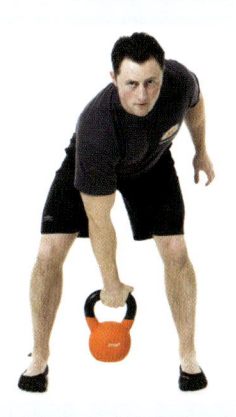

The dead snatch from the hang is performed exactly as with the hang snatch, but with a 1 second pause in the hang position. This will take a lot of the elastic energy out of the lift, challenging the lifting and pulling muscles involved in this exercise more, and will involve a smaller range of motion to generate force than the dead snatch from the floor (exercise 39, page 103).

Exercise 42 Split dead snatch with one kettlebell

This drill is a nice variation of the dead snatch. It takes a little more coordination and is similar to the barbell split snatch exercise that is sometimes adopted by barbell weightlifters. In fact, the barbell split snatch used to be the more popular variation in competitions, but most modern weightlifters prefer the parallel stance variation. This drill is sometimes attempted as more of a swing split snatch, but this doesn't really work very well because of the difficulty in getting back to a parallel stance while the kettlebell is being lowered in the eccentric phase.

Execution
- As in the dead snatch from the floor (exercise 39, page 103), lift the bell from the floor explosively.
- As the bell is in mid-flight after the upwards pull, split the feet and land in a split-stance catch position.
- Briefly hold this catch position and then step forward with the back foot and backwards with the front foot until both feet are parallel again, keeping the kettlebell held overhead.
- Then, lower to the start position and repeat.

Exercise 43 Dead snatch and reverse lunge with one kettlebell

This drill is similar to the split dead snatch, but doesn't involve splitting the legs and dropping the body down in the same position it was in for the lift. This drill can also be performed with a swing variation, rather than the dead start, and is easier to link together than the split snatch. This drill requires good core control, hip stability and a strong core to help decelerate the load. It should only be attempted when the snatch, the split overhead squat and Sagittal plane lunge have been mastered.

Execution
- Start as you would with the split dead snatch (exercise 42, page 105).
- As the bell is pulled upwards, step back with one leg and drop into an overhead split lunge position.
- Briefly hold then step forward and drop the bell back to the start position to repeat.
- Either the same side leg (ipsilateral) or the opposite side leg (contralateral) can be used to lunge backwards for variation.

Exercise 44 Diagonal dead snatch from the floor with one kettlebell

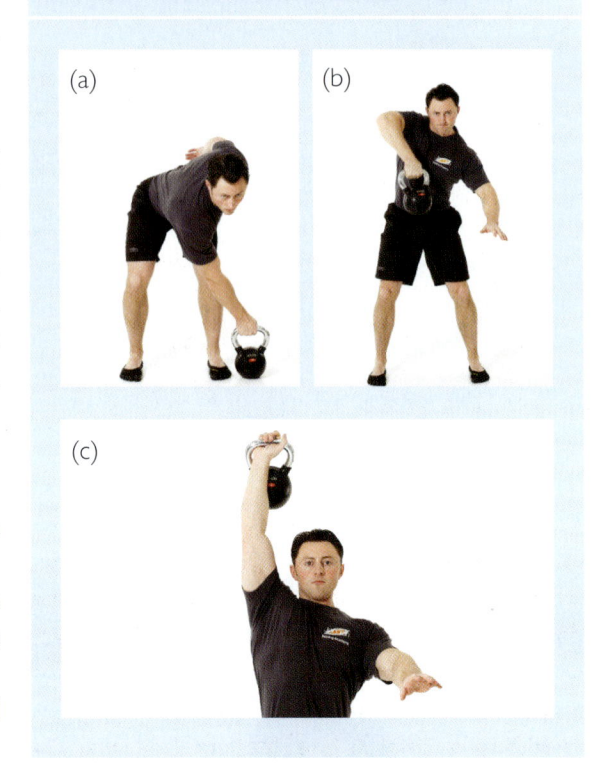

(a)

(b)

(c)

The diagonal dead snatch is only ever performed from the dead position, but in this case the bell rests on the floor to the outside of the opposite leg to the lifting arm. The technique is similar to the dead snatch, but the bell is pulled diagonally across the body into the finish position. This requires more coordination, is more challenging on the posterior core rotators (the glutes and the latissimus dorsi), and requires more frontal plane stabilisation from the shoulder and shoulder girdle musculature for the catch. Do not attempt to undertake this exercise as a continuous swing diagonal snatch as the bell will almost certainly crash into the shin at some point.

Exercise 45 Bottoms up snatch with one kettlebell

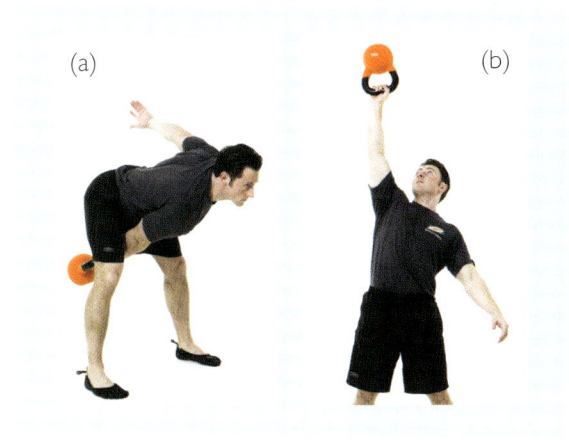

(a) (b)

The bottoms up snatch (see figure 6.3, page 25 for grip position) can be performed from the swing, the hang, from a dead position on the floor or from a dead hang, and it is the catch position that is changed. In this drill there is no punch to the catch phase, rather the kettlebell is caught in the single hand bottoms up position above the head. Many prefer this variation because it does not require the technicalities of the punch phase for the catch of the standard snatch. It will challenge the grip stabilisers, especially if the handle of the bell is quite thick. The bell can be caught with the palm facing forwards, but because of the momentum it tends to flip over in that position. Either catch it at an angle (see exercise 45b) or in a semi-supinated grip with the palm facing inwards.

Exercise 46 Bottoms up snatch with two kettlebells

This is a combination of the swing snatch with two kettlebells and the bottoms up snatch (exercise 45, page 107). Both bells are swung between the legs and then both caught above the head in the bottoms up position. Although an interesting challenge, most people prefer the one hand version so that they can concentrate on catching and holding just one bell above their head at a time.

Exercise 47 Flipped snatch with one kettlebell

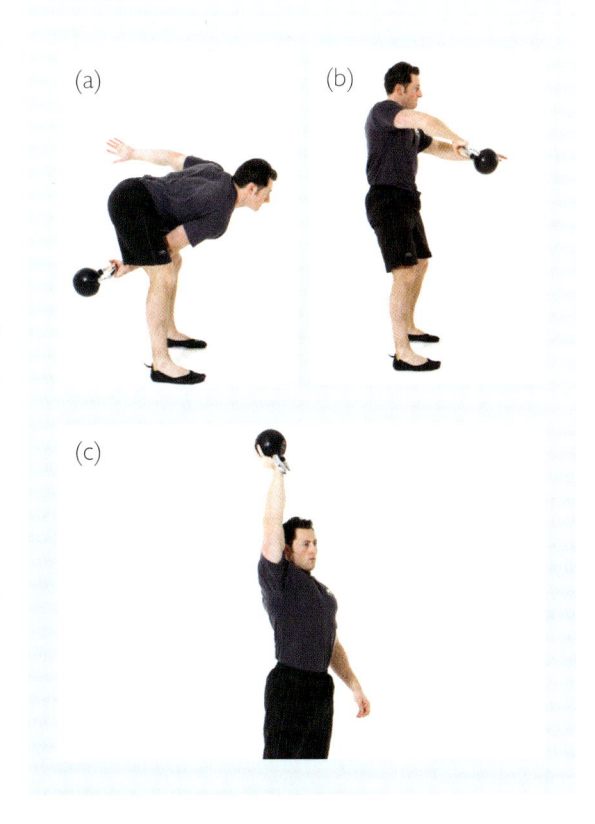

(a) (b)

(c)

The flipped snatch involves releasing the kettlebell after the lift and pull phases and catching the bell part of the kettlebell with a cupped hand and the arm extended. It is actually a great drill to teach the swing snatch to ensure the bell is in the correct place.

Execution
- Perform the swing phase as normal, then extend the hips and pull upwards.
- As the bell follows its normal arc towards the catch position, release the handle of the kettlebell and, allowing the bell to rotate, catch the bell portion in the flipped catch position overhead (exercise 47c). In this position, the handle should be below the bell, next to the wrist or forearm.
- To start the next repetition, cock the wrist and allow the bell to fall forward, catching the handle on the way down.
- Swing between the legs again to repeat.

Exercise variation
As a variation, do not allow the bell to flip in order to catch it. Lift and pull upwards then catch the bell with the handle leading the bell, so that the handle extends outwards and behind the body in the same direction as the fingers.

Exercise 48 Dead snatch with two kettlebells

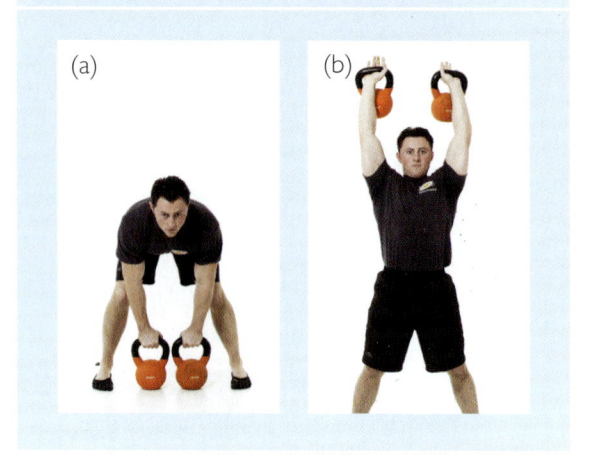

(a)   (b)

With any of the following two kettlebell snatch drills, good coordination and excellent mobility in the thoracic spine and shoulders are required.

Execution
- Start with the bells in line with the heels, shins vertical and posterior chain muscles primed.
- Extend the hips and pull aggressively upwards.
- As the bells travel upwards, punch upwards with both hands to catch the bells above the head.
- Bring back to the start position and repeat.

Exercise 49 (Swing) snatch with two kettlebells

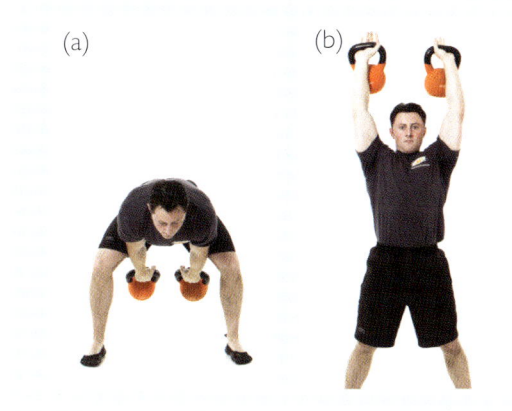

(a) (b)

Execution

This variation involves the swing section as well, rather than starting from a dead start. This will give much needed elastic energy to help elevate both kettlebells above the head in a single action. Have a wider stance to accommodate the two bells for the swing and lean back as the bells drop to ensure they don't pull you forward.

Exercise 50 One hand high pull with release and one kettlebell

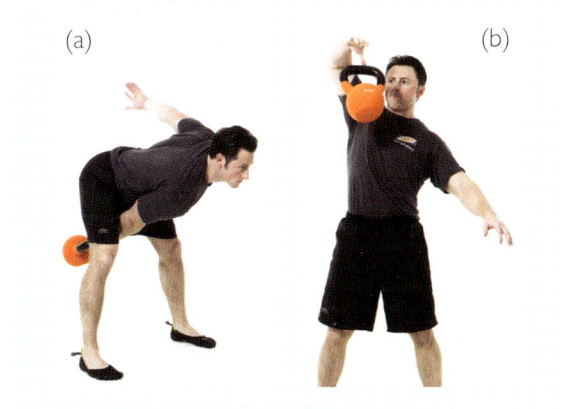

(a) (b)

This can be a handy progression for those individuals not keen on going straight into the flipped snatch.

Execution

- Perform the swing and upwards pull as normal, then, as with the swing and release, just before the top of the arc release the handle.
- If the technique is efficient and smooth, then the bell should stay still. If it wobbles or flips when released, then practise initially just releasing the fingers on the grip of the handle but without fully letting go.
- Once the handle has been released in the full version, follow the bell down as it drops, grip the handle and guide through the legs to commence the next repetition.

SQUAT PATTERN

Exercise 51 Front squat with one kettlebell held in two hands

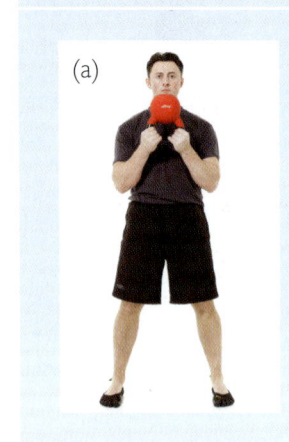

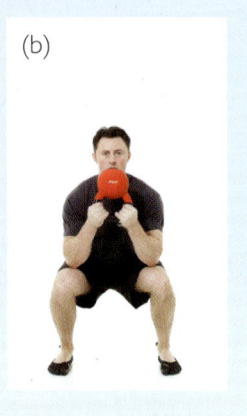

(a) (b)

The front squat is a key exercise for increasing leg strength and endurance as it overloads the quadriceps, hamstrings and calves. It is a fundamental movement pattern, one which is used in everyday life as we move from sitting to standing and vice versa. To achieve a full ROM an adequate amount of ankle flexibility is required, and if this is not possible, it will present as an excessive leaning forwards in the upper body, or an excessive lumbar curve in the spine (lordosis), as well as a reduced depth in the squat pattern. The ideal end point is to have the hamstrings touching the calves, but in many people in the Western world this range is not commonly possible due to an inactive lifestyle.

Aims
The aims of this exercise are to overload the muscles of the legs, in particular the quadriceps; to prepare the body for further squat patterns and to create an adequate ROM for daily functions.

Set-up
- To begin, stand with feet about shoulder width apart but no wider, with the chest upright and the spine and pelvis in neutral position (see chapter 6, page 23).
- Hold the kettlebell in both hands on the horns in a bottoms-up grip.

Execution
- Engage the muscles of the core and bend the knees, keeping the chest upright and the spine in a neutral position (slight curvature in the low back) or flat.
- Keep lowering the hips straight downwards until you reach either a 90-degree position or a full squat position, with the hamstrings touching the calves as preferred.
- Strongly press into the heels to straighten the legs and return to a standing position with the abdominals and glutes contracting.

Exercise 52 Front squat with two kettlebells held in two hands

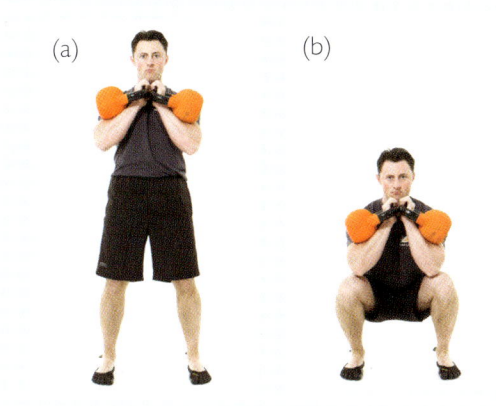

(a) (b)

Using two kettlebells increases the load through the legs, although having an even load also makes the exercise more stable than the usual unilateral version (exercise 17, page 79).

Execution
- Add a second kettlebell, so that you have one in each hand.
- Perform the squat as described in exercise 51.

Exercise 53 Front squat with one kettlebell and bottoms up grip

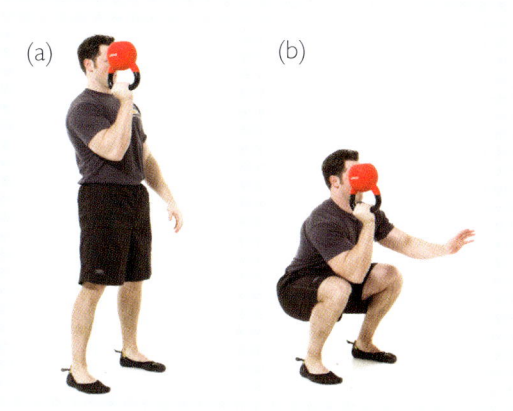

(a) (b)

Execution
- Hold the kettlebell with a single arm bottoms up grip to increase the overload on the muscles of the forearm.
- Perform the squat as described in exercise 51.

Exercise 54 Front squat with two kettlebells in two hands and heels raised

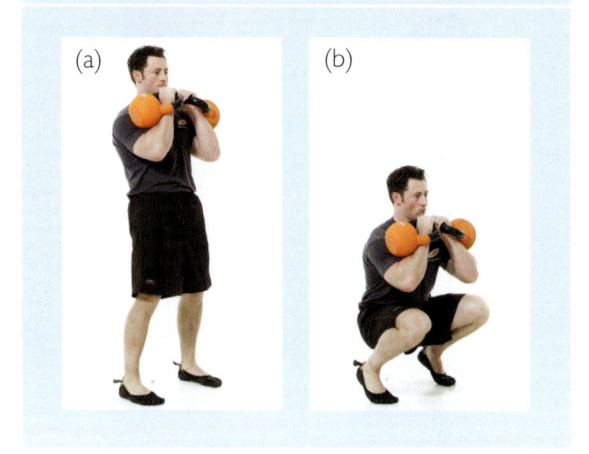

(a) (b)

Exercise 55 Front squat with two kettlebells in two hands and sumo stance

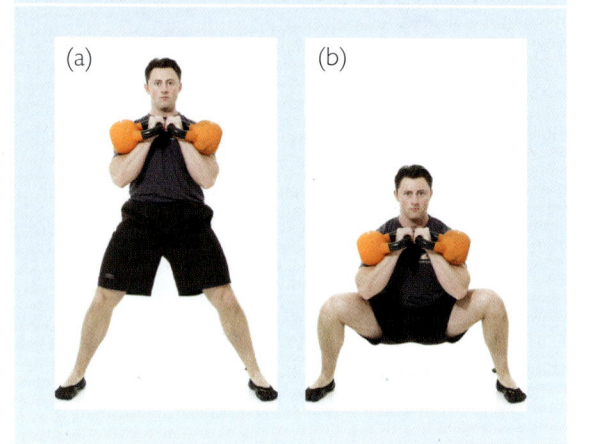

(a) (b)

Execution
- Either perform this drill with heels raised on a wedge, mat or weight plates, or alternatively perform the balance version where the individual deliberately raises the heels and keeps the torso upright.
- Go down to a full depth and briefly hold.
- Then, drive the heels down and straighten the knees to return to standing.

The sumo, or wide, stance recruits the adductors and the quadriceps and requires a more upright torso than the standard front squat. It is a good exercise for those with limited ankle dorsiflexion.

Execution
- Stand in a wide stance with feet pointing out at about 45 degrees and two kettlebells held in a double rack.
- Squat down, keeping a vertical torso, and hold briefly.
- Drive up to the start position and repeat.

Exercise 56 Front squat with two kettlebells in one hand

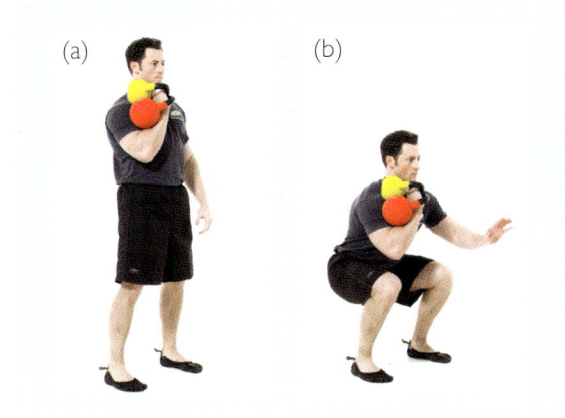

(a) (b)

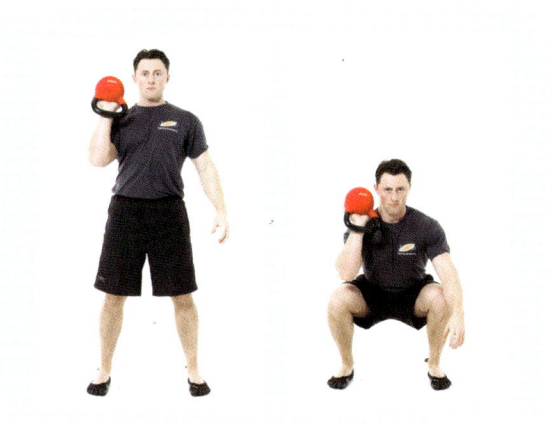

This exercise challenges the gripping muscles of the hand and forearm.

Execution
- Grip both kettlebell handles in the palm of one hand with the two bells stacked one on top of the other.
- Perform the squat as described in exercise 51, page 110.

Exercise 57 Front squat with one kettlebell in one hand and a flipped grip

Execution
- Place the kettlebell in the flipped grip position (see figure 6.4, page 26), with the bell cupped in the palm.
- Keeping the forearm vertical, perform the squat as described in exercise 51, page 110.

Exercise 58 Back squat with one kettlebell in two hands

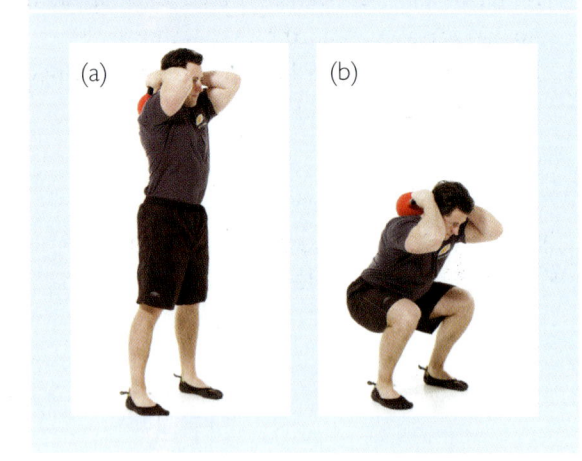

(a) (b)

This is a nice variation from the front squat, utilising a very light load compared to a barbell back squat.

Execution
- Holding the handle with both hands, place the kettlebell on the upper back. *Note*: Do **not** place the kettlebell on the neck.
- Keeping the chest high, perform a full squat technique, as described previously.

Exercise 59 Front squat push press with one kettlebell

This variation combines a front squat and an overhead press. The benefit of this drill is that it makes huge demands on the cardiovascular system, as it is a large compound movement, which requires a great quantity of energy (and thus calorie) expenditure.

Execution
- Holding the bell in the rack position, as you perform the squat pattern and begin to push into the heels to return to a standing position, simultaneously press the kettlebell overhead as you would with a standard one hand overhead press (exercise 18, page 82).
- As you begin to bend the legs, simultaneously lower the kettlebell back to the rack position and repeat.

Exercise 60 Front squat push press with two kettlebells in two hands

This is the two hand variation of the previous drill. It is great for challenging the core and for getting the heart rate up if undertaken for a sustained set.

Execution
- Hold a kettlebell in each hand in the rack position.
- Perform the squat described in exercise 59, using the method of the two hand overhead press.

Exercise 61 Front squat push press with two kettlebells in two hands alternating press

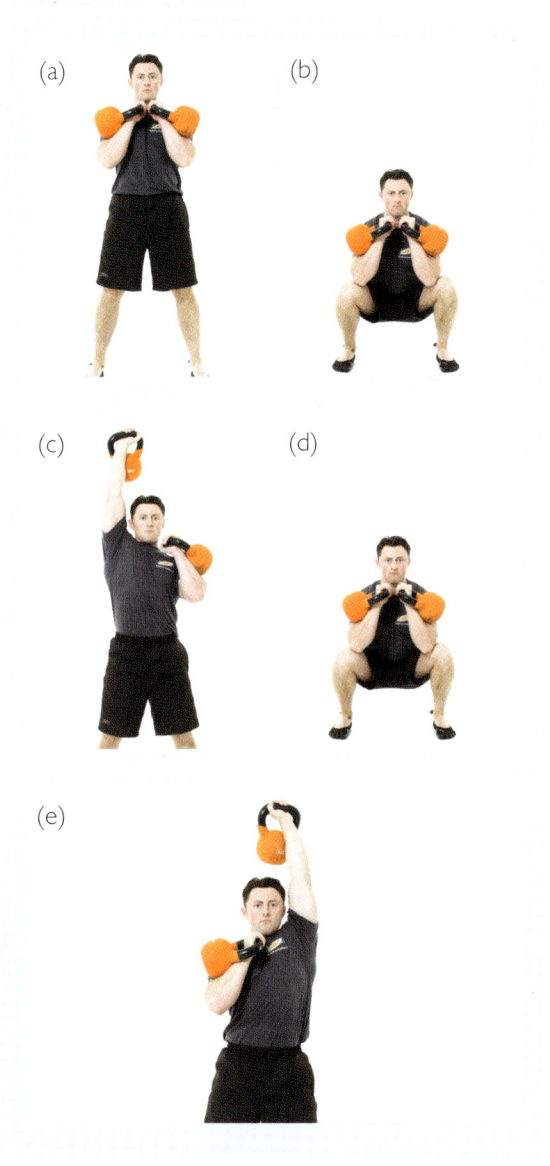

(a) (b)
(c) (d)
(e)

In this variation, perform a single arm press, alternating between the left and right arm.

Execution
- Hold two kettlebells in a double rack.
- Squat down then stand up and press up with one arm to an overhead press position.
- Lower the bell, squat back down, then change arms with each subsequent repetition.

Exercise 62 Single arm overhead squat with one kettlebell

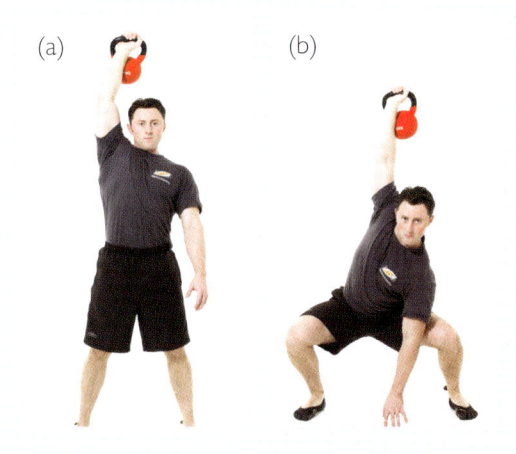

(a) (b)

Execution
- For an overhead squat, ensure an adequate ROM in the shoulders and thoracic spine so that the weight can be lifted overhead without an excessive curve in the lower back.
- For the single arm variation, clean and press or snatch a single kettlebell overhead so that your hand is directly over your shoulder joint and your elbow is locked. *Note*: It is important not to let the elbow bend as you fatigue.
- Stand as if performing a two hand overhead squat with a parallel stance.

- Squat down, keeping a neutral spine with a neutral tracking of the knees over the toes, to either 90 degrees or full depth, keeping the kettlebell directly overhead and positioned between the feet. The body will commonly rotate slightly to accommodate this.

Exercise 63 Single arm overhead squat with one kettlebell and bottoms up or flipped grip

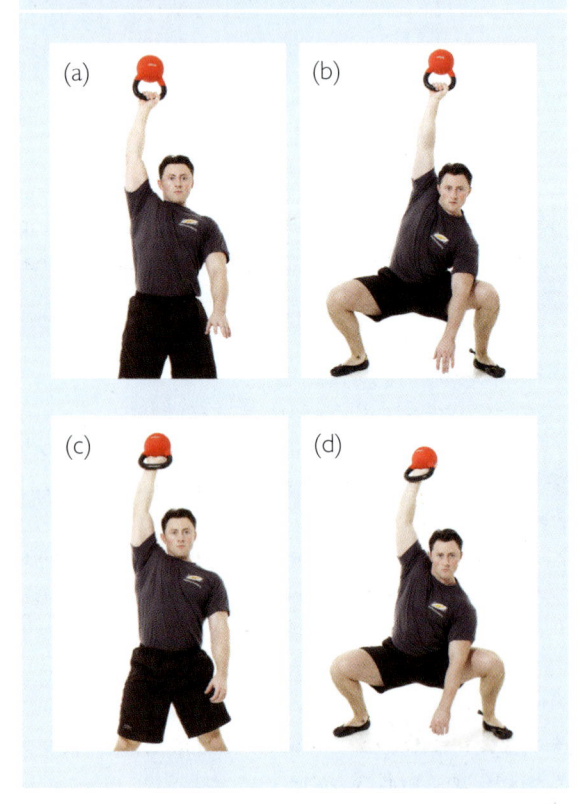

Execution
- Hold the kettlebell in a bottoms up (63a) or flipped grip (63c) position.

- Keeping the arm straight throughout, squat down as low as possible.

Exercise 64 Single arm overhead squat with deadlift and two kettlebells

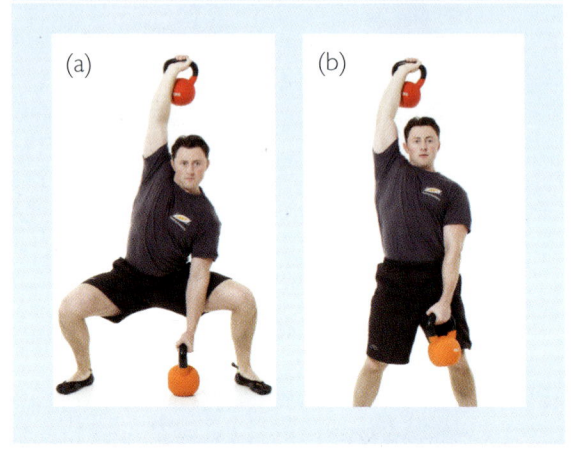

To increase the energy expenditure of the single arm overhead squat an additional weight can be used with the bottom arm.

Execution
- Start with one kettlebell held overhead and one kettlebell positioned between the feet.
- As one arm remains overhead throughout, the other arm holds a weight in between the legs and performs a deadlift action from the floor to hip height as you squat down.
- You can either place the weight on the floor each time to increase the depth of the squat or keep the weight in the hand throughout the deadlift action.

Exercise 65 Squat with one arm overhead and one in rack with two kettlebells

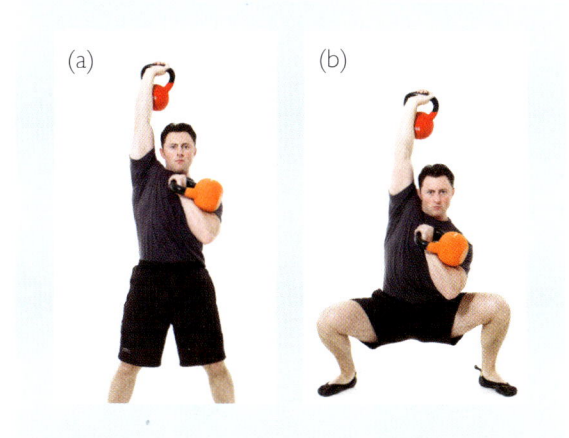

(a) (b)

Exercise 66 Two hand overhead squat with two kettlebells

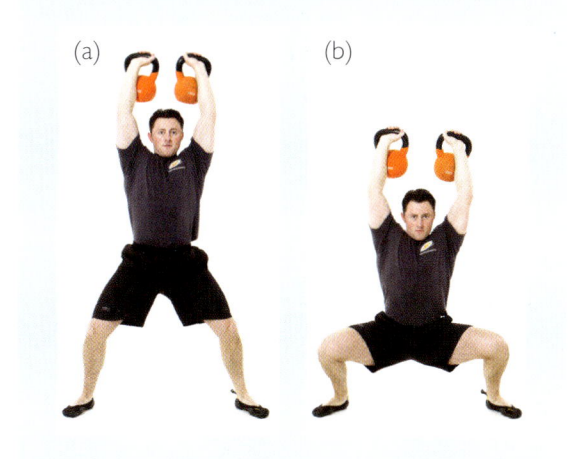

(a) (b)

Execution

- Repeat exercise 64, but hold the second weight in the rack position as the other arm is held overhead. This will allow more load to be used through the legs and will therefore require more stabilising from the core muscles of the hips and stomach.
- You can either place the weight on the floor each time to increase the depth of the squat or keep the weight in the hand throughout the deadlift action.

This variation will overload the shoulders and stabilisers of the lumbar spine and abdominal muscles.

Execution

- Hold two kettlebells, one in each hand.
- Clean and press them overhead so that both bells are held over the shoulders with the elbows locked.
- Hold the kettlebells in line with the shoulders, which will require more control to sustain this position throughout the drill.

Exercise 67 Kettlebell step-up with two kettlebells held at side

A step-up is a functional exercise that allows loading of the legs in a dynamic way, while recruiting the core muscles by the same means as daily movement patterns such as walking or climbing stairs. The intensity of the exercise can be increased by introducing a much higher step, such as a gym bench, or a lower step can be introduced for beginners or those with less control and/or balance.

Set-up
- Stand facing the step you are going to use and have a kettlebell in each arm, with your arms down by your sides.
- Have the palms facing inwards and keep the torso upright with the shoulders relaxed, down and away from the ears.

Execution
- Place one leg on to the step and then transfer your weight into this leg.
- Push strongly down into the foot as you contract the glutes and the abdominal muscles and straighten the top leg.
- Bring the other leg up to stand with the feet together on the step.
- Place the first leg back on to the floor, controlling the descent, and then lower the second leg to return to your starting stance.

Exercise variations
Variations of this exercise include:

- Kettlebell step-up with two kettlebells held in the rack position
- Kettlebell step-up with two kettlebells held overhead
- Kettlebell step-up with two kettlebells held in rack with a press
- Kettlebell lateral step-up with two kettlebells held in rack
- Kettlebell lateral crossover step-up with two kettlebells held in rack
- Kettlebell step-down.

Exercise 68 Kettlebell pistol squat with one kettlebell in rack position

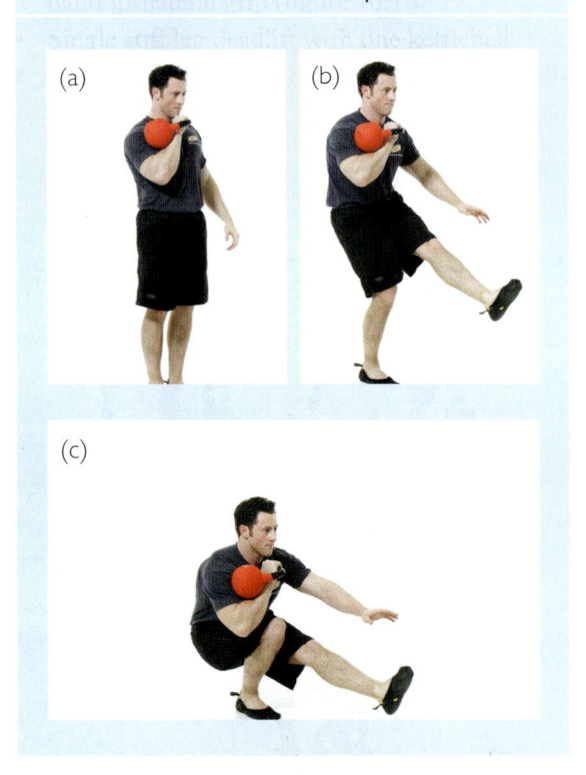

A pistol squat is a challenging asymmetrical exercise that overloads the muscles of the legs. As with other types of squat the ideal ROM is to full depth, with the hamstring touching the calf, but for beginners a smaller ROM can be used initially as balance and leg strength increase with practice.

Aims

The aims of this exercise are to increase the stability of a single leg under load and to increase leg strength through a full ROM.

Execution

- Start by cleaning a single kettlebell to the rack position.
- Stand on one leg with the other leg in front of you and raised just a few inches off the ground. This will provide a counterbalance so that you remain stable.
- Place the second arm on the hip or out at the side for balance.
- It is generally more comfortable for the opposite arm to the working leg to hold the kettlebell, i.e. if you are squatting on the left leg, you would rack the kettlebell on the right arm. However, it can also be held on the same side (see photos).
- Squat down, keeping the heel firmly fixed on the floor and maintaining the position of the front leg straight in front of you. Keep the chest and back upright throughout.
- Ensure that the hips move backwards as the knee simultaneously moves forwards over the toe of the standing leg. Aim to keep the knee tracking over the second or third toe.
- Press the heel down into the floor and contract the glute and thigh of the working leg to drive back up to the start position.

Exercise 69 Kettlebell pistol squat with one kettlebell held in two hands

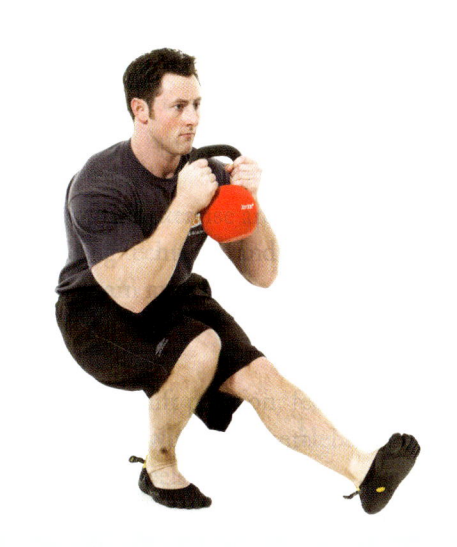

Execution

- Perform this drill as you would exercise 68, but use both hands to hold the kettlebell in the centre of the chest by the handles.
- Keep in mind that there may be additional difficulty, as the other arm cannot be used to stabilise and counter any shifts in the upper body.

Exercise 70 Kettlebell pistol squat with one kettlebell held in two hands extended

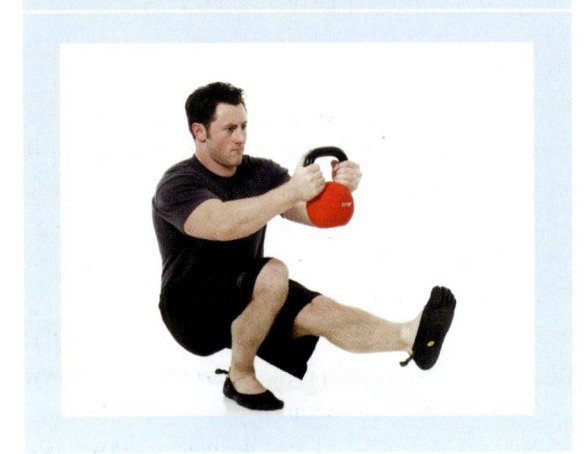

Execution
- For this variation on the pistol squat, hold one kettlebell in both hands out in front of the body.
- Perform the pistol squat.
- This position can be helpful to add stability by counterbalancing the squat action of the lower body. However, holding the weight in this extended position will also increase the fatigue of the shoulders and arms.

Exercise 71 Kettlebell pistol squat with two kettlebells in the rack position

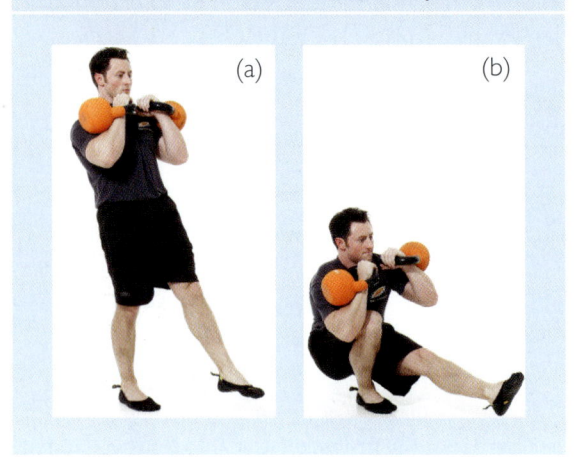

(a) (b)

Execution
- Hold one kettlebell in each hand in rack position. This will allow you to increase the weight load through the legs once you have mastered the stability aspect.
- Perform the pistol squat as you would for exercise 68.

Exercise 72 Kettlebell split squat with two kettlebells in the rack position

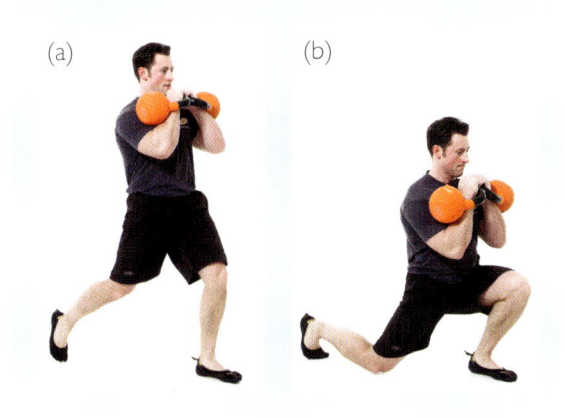

(a)   (b)

Split squats create an asymmetrical load through the legs and muscles of the obliques and lower back, which means they have excellent crossover to any sport that involves walking or running actions. Because of the asymmetry of the exercise, any weaknesses or muscle imbalances will present. Commonly those who are restricted through the front of the body, especially the hip flexors and quads, find this exercise really difficult and tend to lean too far forwards to compensate, shortening these restricted muscles. Foam roller work to release the front of the thighs or dynamic stretches specifically for the hip flexors can be performed to help address this.

A weakness in the stabilisers of the hips, or anywhere along the chain of muscles comprising the posterior sling system will present as the hips being unable to maintain a horizontal position. Focusing on contracting the glutes and core and on keeping the hips level may help to reduce this, otherwise isolation exercises may be required to strengthen the glutes in the long term.

Aims

The aims of this exercise are to progress from a parallel stance to an asymmetrical stance and to overload the legs with a less stable stance.

Execution

- Clean the kettlebells to the double rack position then take a big step forwards so that there is about a leg's length between the front and back foot. Those with tight hip flexors will likely, and unknowingly, take a shorter step to compensate for their restrictions.
- Keep the toes of both feet tracking straight forwards as this will ensure correct recruitment of the muscles of the hips.
- Keep the front heel firmly fixed on the floor throughout and the back foot balanced on the ball of the foot.
- Keeping the hips as level as possible, bend the front knee to reach at least 90 degrees of flexion, ensuring the patella tracks over the second or third toe. Keep the torso upright throughout the movement, so that the chest and back leg are in line.
- Extend the front leg back up to the start position and repeat.

Exercise variations

Other split squat variations include:

- Kettlebell split squat with one kettlebell held in ipsilateral rack
- Kettlebell split squat with one kettlebell held in contralateral rack
- Kettlebell split squat with two kettlebells held by the sides
- Kettlebell split squat with two kettlebells held overhead

- Kettlebell split squat press with one kettlebell held in contralateral rack
- Kettlebell split squat with two kettlebells held in rack with rear foot raised
- Kettlebell split squat with two kettlebells held in rack with front foot raised.

Exercise 73 Kettlebell lunge Sagittal plane with two kettlebells in the rack position

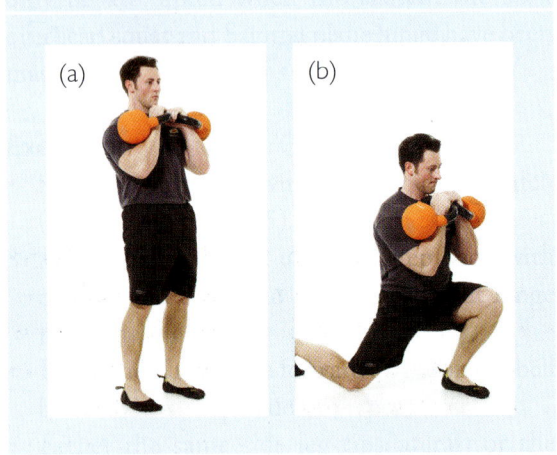

(a) (b)

Once the static split squat has been mastered it can be progressed to a dynamic lunge.

Execution
- With the split squat the legs remain fixed in the split stance throughout the movement, whereas for the lunge variation you need to start with feet together and then take a big step forwards.
- Control the descent then strongly push through the heel of the front leg to return the foot back to the starting position with both feet together.
- Because of the dynamic nature of this exercise any weaknesses will quickly present. Focus on keeping the front foot always pointing forwards and the hips level. Keep the movement fluid and controlled as much as possible.

Exercise 74 Kettlebell lunge frontal plane with two kettlebells in the rack position

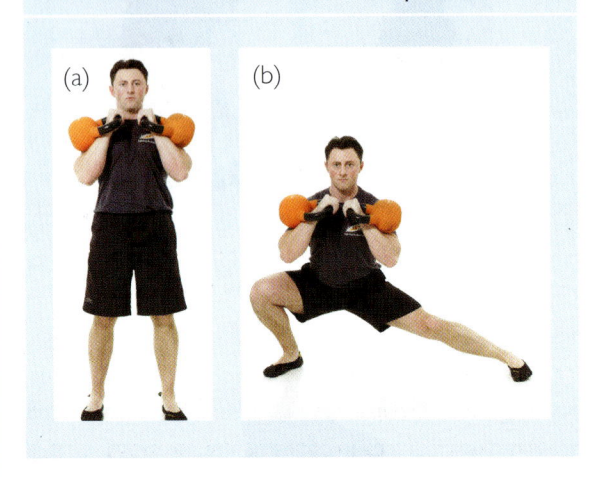

(a) (b)

To work the body in the frontal plane a lateral lunge can be performed.

Execution
- Rack the kettlebells, one in each hand, and stand with the feet together in neutral or up to 20–30 degrees of external rotation.
- Keeping the hips square to the front, take a big step out to the side allowing the foot to naturally turn out, while keeping an upright torso to maintain the position of the kettlebells.
- Lunge down into the working leg, keeping the other leg straight with both feet flat on the floor.
- Extend the working leg strongly to bring the two feet back together.
- This exercise can be performed alternating the right and left leg or as a single set on one side.

Exercise 75 Kettlebell crossover lunge frontal plane with two kettlebells in the rack position

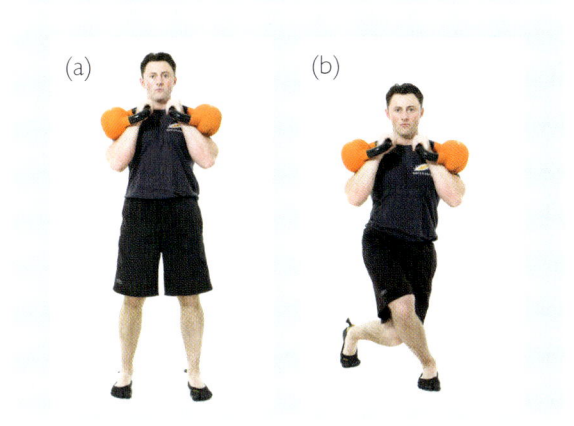

(a) (b)

Exercise 76 Kettlebell crossover lunge frontal plane with two kettlebells, one in rack and one by the side

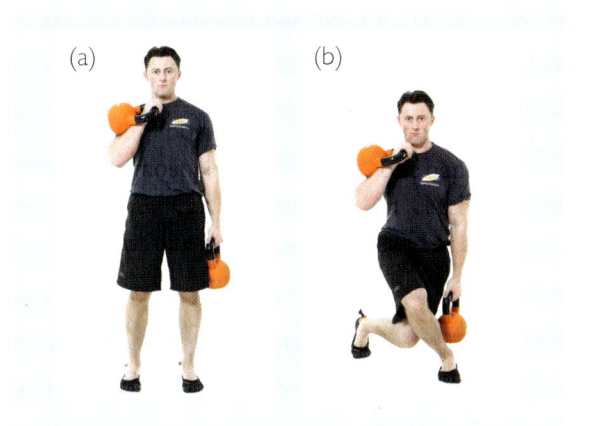

(a) (b)

Execution

- For this variation on exercise 74, step one leg over the other to perform a lateral lunge across the body, i.e. step the right leg in front of the left leg, bending both legs at the end range.
- The benefit of this is a greater increase in the activation of the abductors on the hips.

Execution

- For this drill, have one kettlebell in rack and hold one kettlebell by the side of the body.
- Hold the kettlebell by the side on the contralateral side and lower to the front foot to overload the hip abductors of the lead leg.
- Perform the lunge as you would for exercise 74.

Exercise variations

Other lunge variations include:

- Kettlebell lunge Sagittal backward with two kettlebells in the rack position
- Kettlebell lunge Sagittal walking with two kettlebells in the rack position
- Kettlebell lunge Sagittal forward with rotation with two kettlebells in the rack position
- Kettlebell lunge Sagittal forward with press with two kettlebells in the rack position.

PRESS PATTERN

Overhead presses with the kettlebell require an extensive ROM in the shoulders. A reduction here presents as an excessive lumbar curve arching in the lower back as the arms are raised overhead, commonly from about 90 degrees and above. If an individual does not have the required flexibility to perform this drill, they will not only excessively work the lower back but the shoulders will not be able to effectively produce force in good alignment either. If this is the case, it is advisable to spend some time improving the ROM before attempting the overhead lifts. Many of the other drills will work the shoulders to some extent, as part of a compound movement anyway, but in a way that will not increase your risk of injury or further restriction.

For those who have sufficient movement, the overhead drills recruit the core muscles as you stabilise a heavy load above the body, and can require grip and shoulder strength. Always start with a conservative weight, as you don't want to risk dropping a heavy kettlebell on your head or on anyone else either!

Exercise 77 Two hand press with two kettlebells

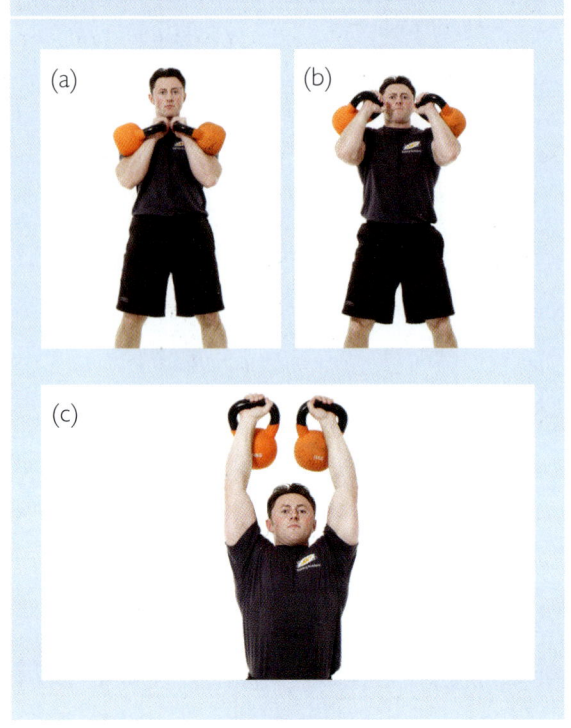

(a) (b) (c)

Aims

The aims of this exercise are to overload the muscles of the deltoid muscles of the shoulders, the triceps and the stabilisers of the shoulders (the rotator cuff and latissimus dorsi) and to overload the muscles of the core through stabilising a load overhead.

Set-up

- Stand in a strong parallel stance with the feet around hip width or slightly wider.
- Start with the kettlebells (one in each hand) in rack position.
- Engage the core muscles and ensure a neutral spine before you start so that the pelvis is in neutral and the torso is upright.

Execution

- Perform the press style that feels most efficient for you (either out to the side or straight upwards), rotating the hands to finish with the palms facing forwards and the elbows locked.
- Keep the glutes contracted so that the pelvis doesn't tilt forwards or backwards, and the abdominal muscles braced to stabilise the load overhead.
- To return to the rack position draw the elbows downwards and be aware of a sensation of pulling the bell downwards under control.

Exercise 78 Alternating two hand press with two kettlebells

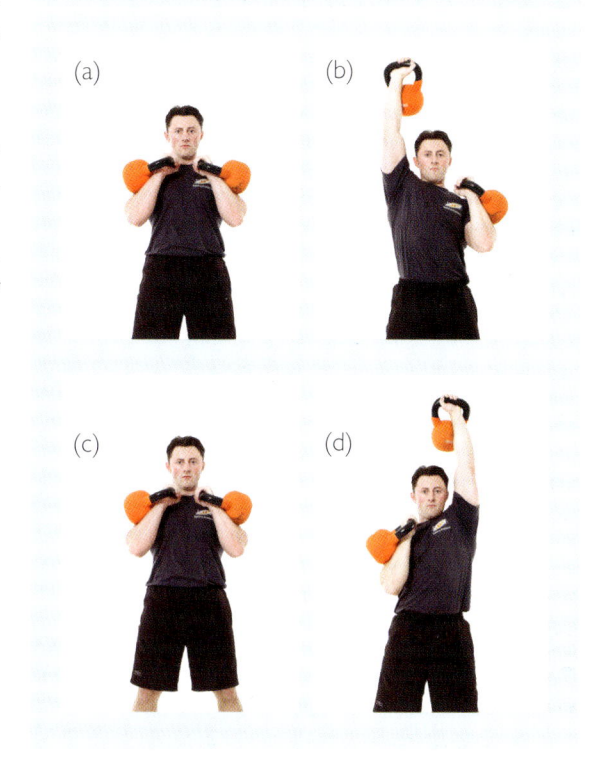

(a) (b)

(c) (d)

As you alternate moving one arm, the body is stabilised through the asymmetrical load on the core muscles.

Execution

- As with the two hand press (exercise 77), start by holding two kettlebells in the rack position in the same stance.
- In this variation, alternate pressing the kettlebells overhead one at a time, fully re-racking one kettlebell before beginning the press action of the other arm. You may also be able to press a heavier weight by isolating the press to a single arm at a time in this way.

Exercise 79 Alternating two hand press with two kettlebells (or see saw press)

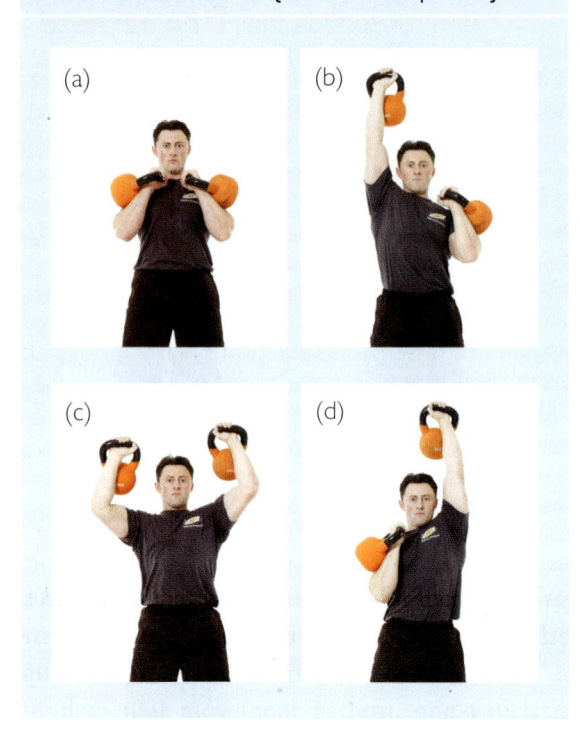

(a) (b)
(c) (d)

This exercise gives a great overload on the cardiovascular system and creates a high demand on the core muscles to stabilise in an asymmetrical movement pattern at a dynamic pace.

Execution
- As with exercise 78, alternately press the right and left arms.
- Rather than completing each rack before lifting the opposing arm, in this variation create a 'see-saw' effect by beginning the next shoulder press as the first arm is lowering to create a continuous alternate pressing action.

Exercise 80 One hand press with one kettlebell in a flipped grip

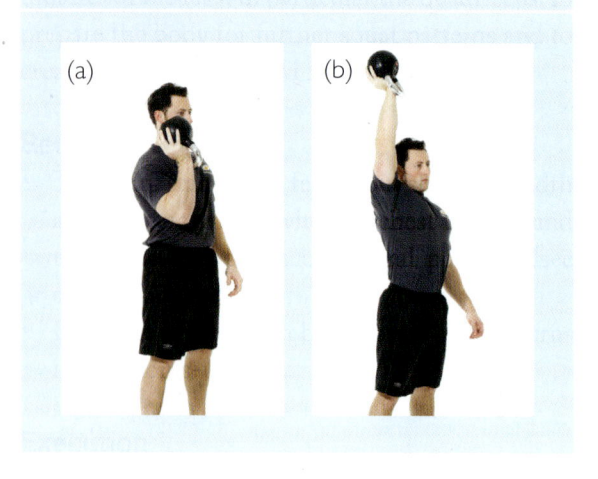

(a) (b)

Execution
- Holding the bell in the cupped palm of the flipped grip (see figure 6.4, page 26), press it upwards to a full locked position.
- This provides a slight variation to the standard grip adopted for most pressing drills.

Exercise 81 One hand press with one kettlebell in a bottoms up press

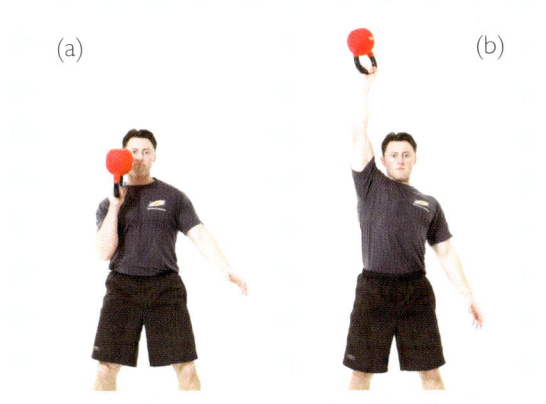

(a)   (b)

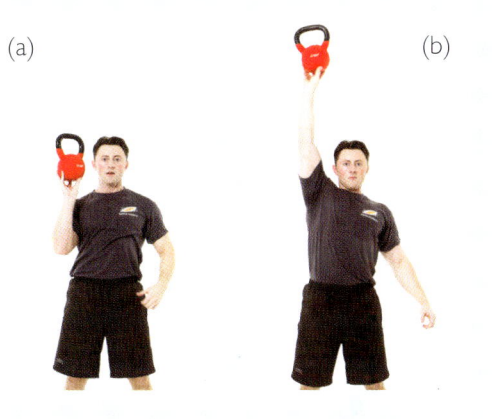

This is a great exercise for challenging the gripping muscles of the hand and forearm.

Execution
- Start in the bottoms up clean position, also known as the pistol grip (figure 6.3, page 25).
- Press the bell upwards, keeping the handle directly underneath the bell at all times to prevent it from flipping over.

Exercise 82 One hand press with one kettlebell in a fingertip hold

(a)   (b)

Fingergrip variations were apparently popular with Victorian strongman Arthur Saxon, and will help to develop strength in the fingers, just like performing press-ups on the fingertips.

Execution
- Balance the bell on the fingertips, then press up to the locked position as normal.
- Return to starting position and repeat.

Exercise variations
Other variations of these drills include:

- One hand press with two kettlebells in one hand
- Two hand alternating press in bottoms up grip

Exercise 83 Overhead press with rotation and one kettlebell

(a) (b)

(c)

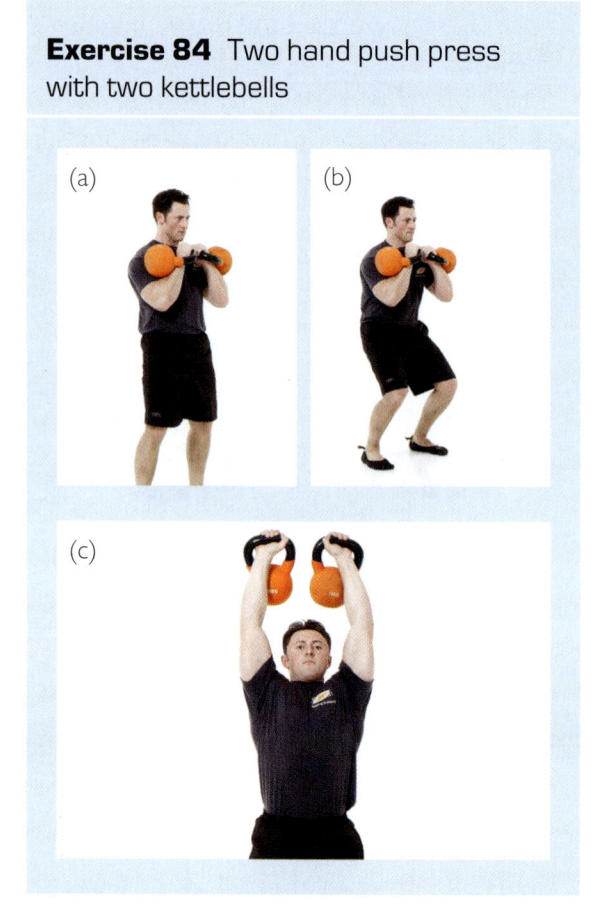

Exercise 84 Two hand push press with two kettlebells

(a) (b)

(c)

This exercise can also be performed with two kettlebells being pressed or with an alternating press with rotation.

Execution
- With one kettlebell in rack, press the bell up above the head as normal.
- In this variation, rotate the torso at the same time as you press the bell, away from the side you are pressing.
- Feet can be kept flat on the floor, but many will prefer to lift the heel up on the ipsilateral side for comfort.

The push press is designed to use the elastic energy from the lower body dip and drive to generate more force to lift the weight up. This variation will recruit the muscles of the upper and lower body and will promote good coordination between the two. It can also be performed with one kettlebell. Always push press with a heavier kettlebell than the weight used for the standard press.

Execution
- Starting from a parallel stance, with two kettlebells in rack position, bend the legs into a

semi-squat position to load up the muscles of the legs.
- Then immediately straighten the legs and use the energy to lift the bells off the chest, pressing overhead for the final phase until the elbow is locked out.
- Lower the weight to rack, pause, then bend the legs again for the next repetition.

Exercise 85 Two hand split jerk with two kettlebells

For the jerk exercise the weight of the kettlebells should be either heavier, or more volume (repetitions) should be achieved. This is because the jerk is biomechanically more efficient than the press or the push press.

Execution
- The jerk follows the same the process as the push press, with the dip and drive upwards, but instead of the press to finish the movement, the body should drop down to catch the kettlebells with arms locked.
- Because the kettlebells are projected upwards through the drive of the hips and thighs and then caught with the arms already locked, there is minimal involvement of the arms, hence the greater efficiency over a standard press or push press.
- As the kettlebells are moving upwards, separate the legs into a split stance catch position. Ensure the rear leg is straighter than a standard lunge for increased stability.
- Once caught, push back with the front foot and slide the rear foot forward until both feet are under the hips in a parallel stance.

Exercise 86 Two hand power jerk with two kettlebells

The two hand power jerk is one of the key exercises to perfect for those looking to compete in Girevoy Sport, since it forms part of both the biathlon (two hand two kettlebell jerk) and the long cycle (two kettlebell clean and jerk), two of the major disciplines in the competitive sport.

Execution
- The technique is the same as the split jerk (exercise 85), except the legs are not split and the bells are caught in a parallel stance overhead squat position.

- This is the preferred technique for competitions simply because there is less energy expended by not moving the feet. The split jerk is more commonly used in barbell weightlifting where the load is heavier and only one repetition is performed.

Exercise 87 One hand side press with one kettlebell

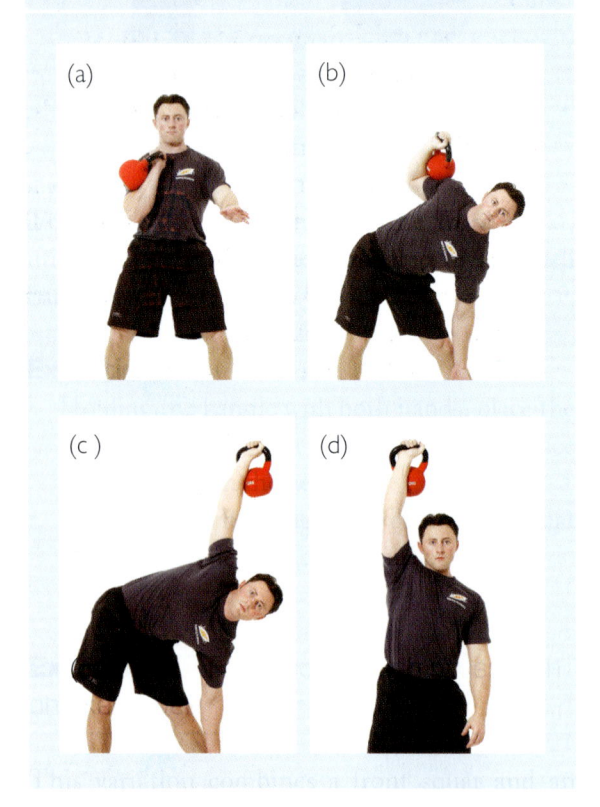

(a) (b) (c) (d)

The one hand side press with one kettlebell is a strength and stability exercise, grouped under the press movement pattern, and is a progression from the windmill (see exercise 20, page 89).

Aims

The aims of this exercise are to increase frontal plane stability while overhead lifting and to work the lateral core, hip stabilisers and pressing muscles. This exercise is best performed over low repetitions and with a heavy weight, just as the strongmen of the early 1900s performed it.

Execution

- Clean the kettlebell up to the rack position.
- In a standing position, inhale and brace then rotate the arm outwards.
- Start with the kettlebell held out to the side at shoulder height with the elbow on the latissimus dorsi.
- Rotate the feet 30 degrees keeping heels on the same line. Push the rear hip over the rear foot and bend front knee slightly.
- Press your body under the kettlebell as you slide the back of the hand down the inner thigh and lower leg.
- Perform the lowering part of a windmill while at the same time pressing the bell upwards. Focus on pressing the body down underneath the kettlebell, rather than just lifting the weight. Focus the eyes on a point of the ceiling throughout.
- When the arm is locked, use the lateral core and hip abductors to perform the concentric phase of the windmill to bring the body to an upright position.
- Lower the kettlebell and repeat.

Exercise 88 One hand bent press with one kettlebell

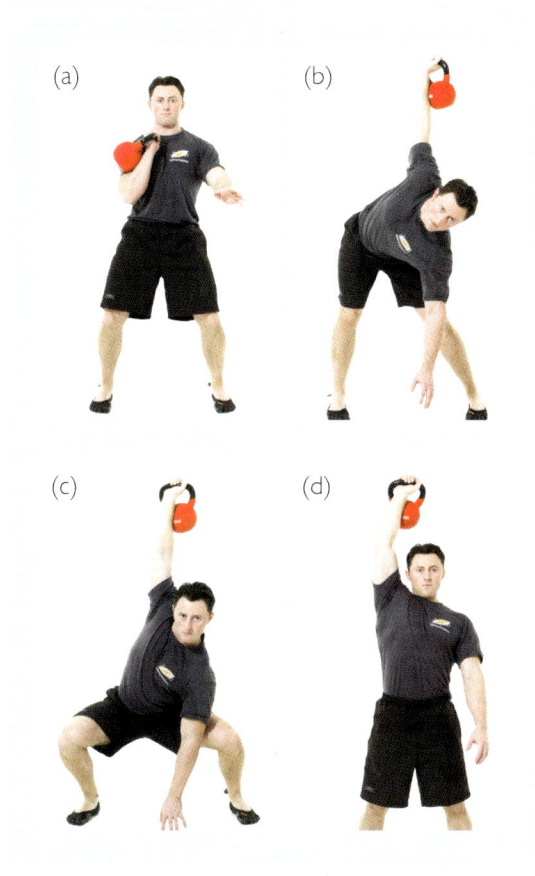

(a) (b)
(c) (d)

The bent press is a strength and stability exercise and is a variation from the side press, which enables you to lift heavy loads over the head.

Aims
The aims of this exercise are to increase frontal and transverse plane stability while overhead lifting and to work the lateral core, hip stabilisers and pressing muscles.

Execution
- Clean the kettlebell up to the rack position.
- In a standing position, inhale and brace.
- Press the kettlebell upwards and rotate the torso under the bell and downwards.
- Support the other arm on the thigh to take some of the load off the spine and focus your eyes on the kettlebell throughout.
- When the arm is locked, squat down and then push up into a standing position.
- Lower the kettlebell and repeat.

Exercise 89 Two hand anyhow with two kettlebells

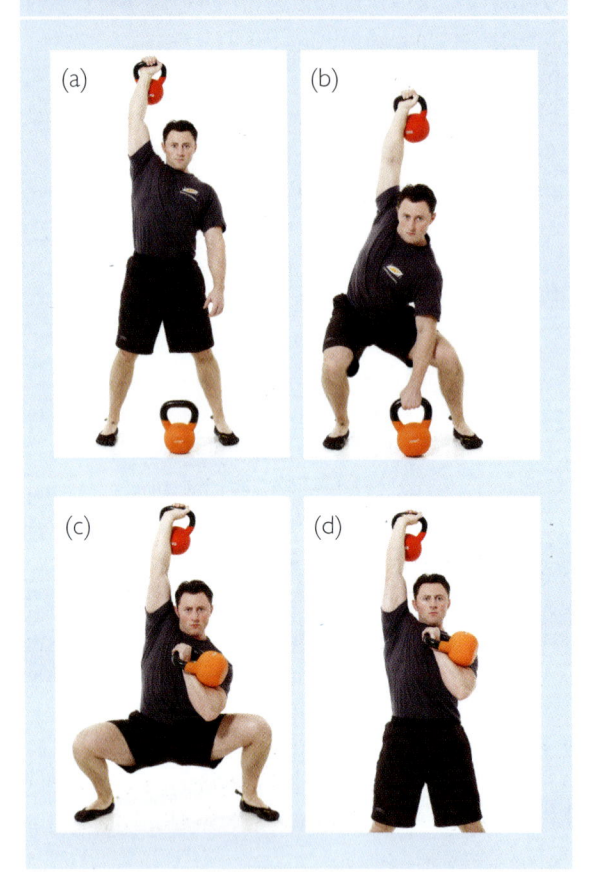

(a) (b) (c) (d)

Execution
- Perform a clean and jerk, a snatch, a side press or a bent press with one kettlebell.
- With the other arm resting on the thigh/knee of the front leg, squat down and pick up the second kettlebell by the handle and curl it to the shoulder or bring the shoulder to the kettlebell.
- Stand up with the second kettlebell in the rack position then press/jerk it overhead.
- Lower both of the kettlebells and repeat.
- As an alternative, lift the second kettlebell up to rack by using more of a windmill-style technique – hold the first kettlebell above the head and reach down to pick up the second. Then, curl it off the inner thigh and use the core to get to a standing position. Either style is acceptable and it is worth practising both.
- Perform with heavy loads and low repetitions.

This exercise, as the name suggests, allows an individual to lift one kettlebell overhead and then a second weight by their preferred method. It is an old school strength and stability exercise and is a progression from the side press or bent press, enabling an individual to lift two heavy loads above the head.

Exercise 90 Floor press with two kettlebells

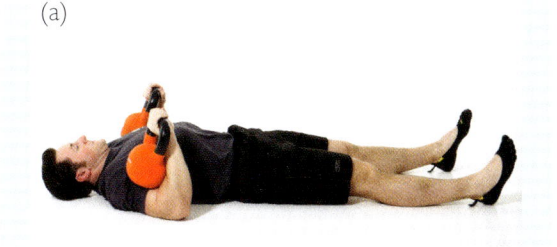

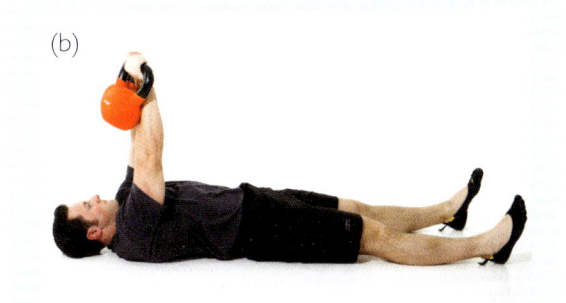

(a)

(b)

Exercise 91 Bridge press with two kettlebells

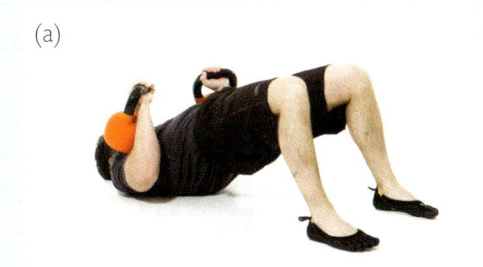

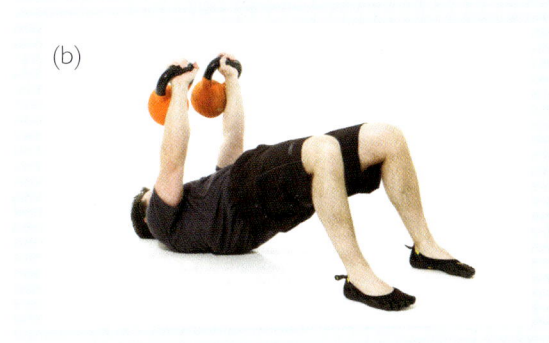

(a)

(b)

The floor press is a kettlebell variation of the barbell bench press, but is performed on the floor. Although working the chest with this type of horizontal pressing motion is deemed by many as paramount to their training programme, it is but a small part and is insignificant in comparison with kettlebell drills such as the snatch, windmill, Turkish get-up, clean and jerk.

Execution
- Lie supine with the legs straight and the kettlebells pressed up vertically.
- Bend the elbows down to the sides until just before they touch the floor.
- Pause briefly, then extend the arms to press the weights upwards.

Execution
- Start as you would the floor press (exercise 90).
- Lift the hips off of the ground into a supine bridge position.
- Press the kettlebells upwards, pause briefly, then bring them back to the sides.

Exercise 92 Alternating bridge press with two kettlebells

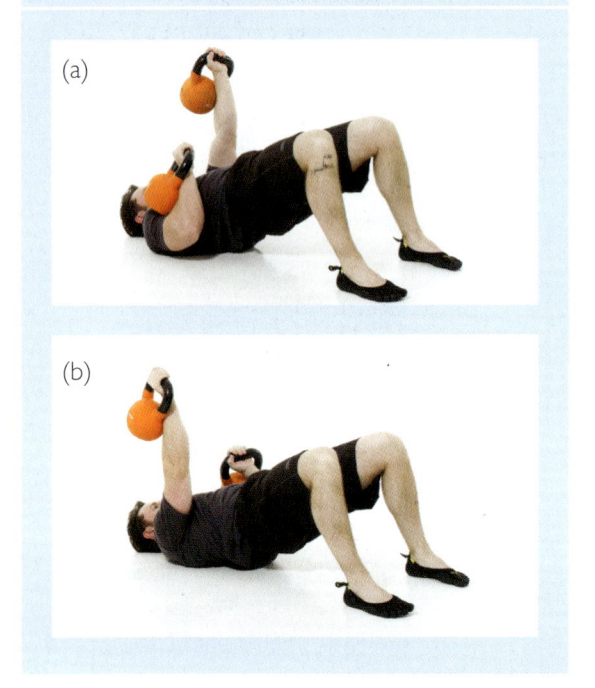

(a)

(b)

Exercise 93 One hand sots press with two kettlebells

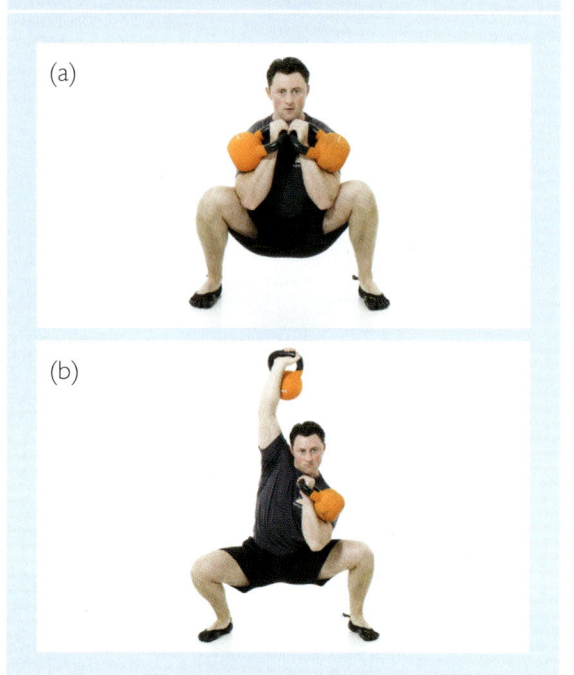

(a)

(b)

Execution
- Start as you would the floor press (exercise 90, page 133).
- Lift the hips off of the ground into a supine bridge position.
- Press the kettlebells upwards, alternating pressing with the left and right arm and bringing them back to the sides.
- A further variation to this exercise is the alternating wrestler's bridge press. Instead of bridging on the upper back, the individual bridges on the head. It is an exercise used by wrestlers and mixed martial artists to improve neck strength for their sports.

This drill really challenges shoulder mobility and stability and is a great remedial drill to improve strength in the overhead squat position.

Execution
- Clean two kettlebells into the rack position and squat down into a full front squat position.
- Holding this position, press one kettlebell up until the arm is fully extended, keeping the bell positioned over the feet.
- Bring the kettlebell back down and repeat on both sides.

Exercise variations
To vary this exercise, press two kettlebells together or with an alternating press pattern.

Exercise 94 Side plank press

(a)

(b)

- From this position brace the core and, keeping the torso completely still, press the kettlebell upwards until a locked arm position is reached.
- Briefly hold then lower to the start position and repeat.

Exercise 95 Press-up with kettlebells

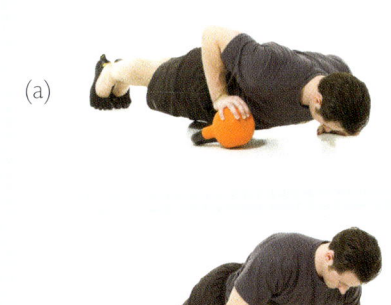

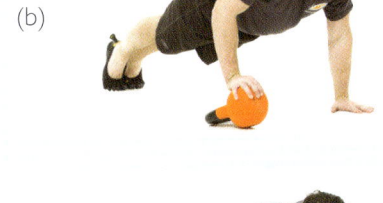

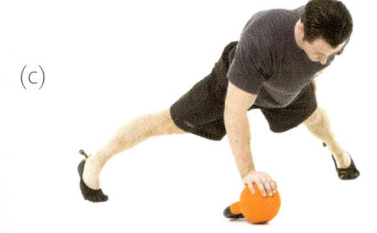

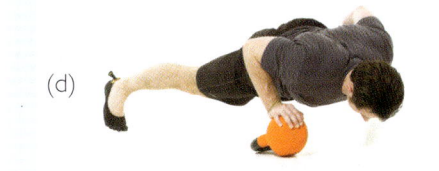

(a)

(b)

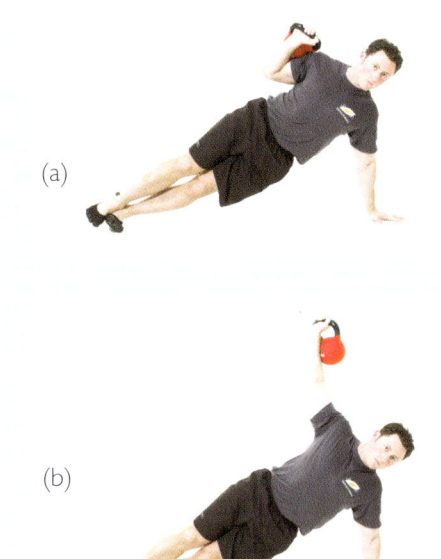

(c)

(d)

The side plank press is a stepping stone exercise towards completing the standing side press.

Execution
- Adopt a lateral or side plank position with the feet on top of each other (see photos) or with one foot in front of the other for more stability.
- Lift the kettlebell from the floor and rotate the arm out so that the elbow is resting on the latissimus dorsi. The body can be held on the hand with the arm extended (as shown), which will require more shoulder stability, or on the elbow and forearm.

(e)

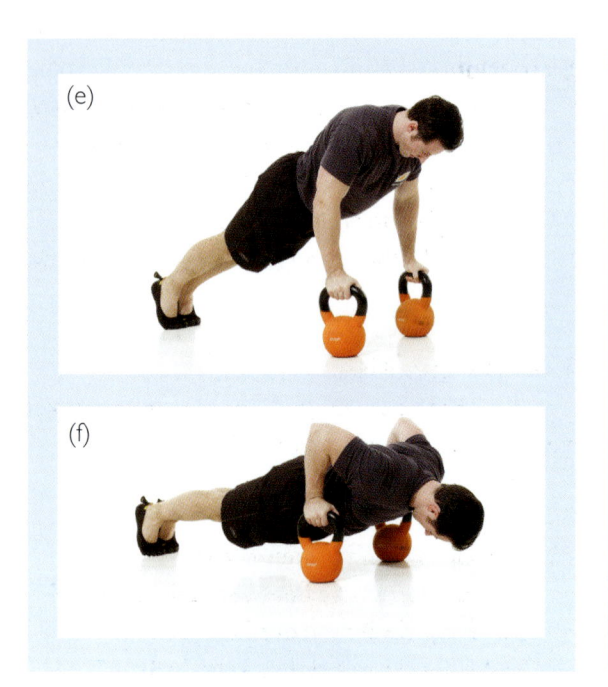

(f)

PULL PATTERN

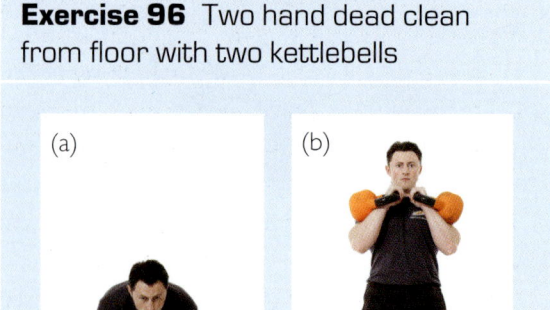

Exercise 96 Two hand dead clean from floor with two kettlebells

(a)

(b)

There are a variety of standard press-up drills that can be adopted for use with kettlebells. Many of these drills are traditionally undertaken on medicine balls, but the kettlebell makes a nice change as they don't move anywhere near as much as a medicine ball. The photos below show the press-up with one hand on the kettlebell (a and b); the single hand press up on kettlebell (c and d) and a balance press-up on two kettlebells (e and f).

This is one of the key kettlebell drills to master since it requires the individual to be able to pick the kettlebells up from the floor safely and effectively to the rack position. This particular exercise is a posterior-chain strength and power combination exercise, which works the lift and pull patterns to bring the kettlebells to the shoulder.

Set-up
- Begin in the deadlift position, feet shoulder width apart with the kettlebells positioned between the heels on the floor.
- Brace the core to stabilise and protect the back.
- Limit knee bend to adequately load the posterior chain.

Execution
- Extend the hips and knees forcefully and aggressively, then pull upwards.

- As the kettlebells accelerate upwards, perform a double uppercut punch upwards to the centre of the chest with both arms to flip the handles around the bells. Keep the fingers positioned 'inside' the handles to avoid 'pinching'. The bells should rest on the forearms with the arms held diagonally across the chest and ribs (the rack position).
- Twist the thumbs forwards to flip the bells over and guide backwards through the legs back to the start position and repeat.
- Keep the repetitions low when learning the technique and gradually build up the volume.

Exercise 97 Two hand (swing) clean with two kettlebells

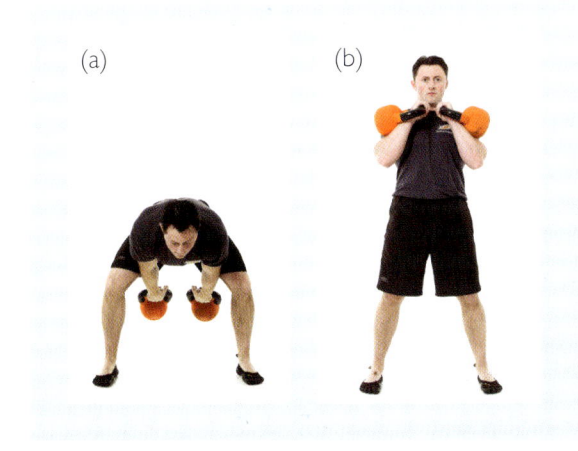

(a)   (b)

This exercise forms part of the long cycle discipline in kettlebell competitions.

Execution
- Adopt a slightly wider-than-normal clean stance to accommodate the two kettlebells.
- Perform one or two double kettlebell swings, then clean up to the double rack position.
- Briefly hold then swing between the legs and repeat.

Exercise variations
Other variations, integrations or progressions involving the clean exercise include:

- Hang clean with one kettlebell
- Hang clean with two kettlebells
- Dead clean from the floor with one kettlebell
- Dead hang clean with one kettlebell
- Dead hang clean with two kettlebells
- Long cycle press (clean and press) with one kettlebell
- Long cycle press (clean and press) with two kettlebells
- Long cycle jerk (clean and jerk) with one kettlebell
- Long cycle jerk (clean and jerk) with two kettlebells
- Long cycle squat (clean and squat) with one kettlebell
- Long cycle squat (clean and squat) with two kettlebells
- Long cycle squat push press (clean and squat push press) with one kettlebell
- Long cycle squat push press (clean and squat push press) with two kettlebells.

Exercise 98 Alternating cleans with two kettlebells

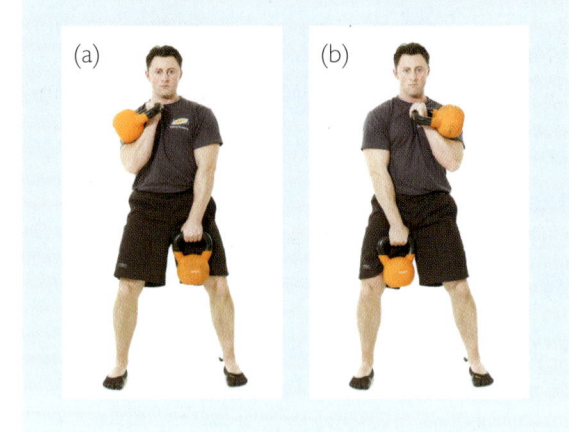

(a)   (b)

Exercise 99 Bottoms up clean with one kettlebell

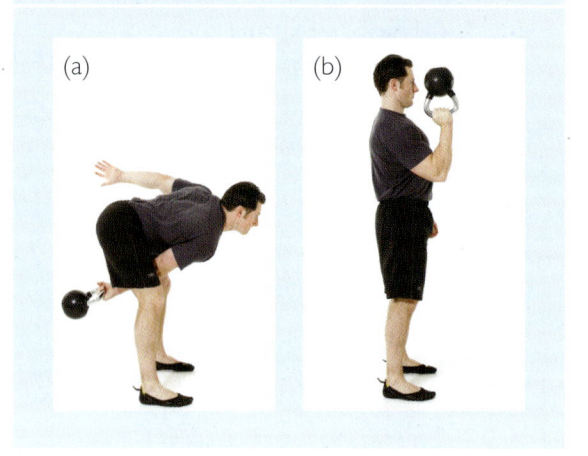

(a)   (b)

Performing alternating snatches is quite awkward, so is not really recommended as a comfortable exercise to do. Alternating cleans is much more comfortable and so is a more widely used variation of the two hand clean drills. This particular exercise is performed more as an alternating hang clean rather than the swing variation.

Execution
- With both kettlebells in the rack position, drop one down between the legs to about knee height, then immediately change direction and clean back up to the rack.
- Change kettlebells and repeat.
- Keep an upright torso position and do not lean forward too much or it will be difficult to hold the racked kettlebell in place.

The bottoms up clean, or pistol grip clean as it is also known, is one of my favorite drills for improving in the swing clean exercise, as well as increasing grip strength.

Execution
- Swing the kettlebell between the legs then extend the hips and catch the kettlebell above the vertical forearm in the bottoms up position.
- Squeeze the handle tightly to ensure the bell does not flip over.
- Briefly hold then swing between the legs again and repeat.

Exercise variations
As a progression, add some of the following bottoms up drills within your programme:

- Bottoms up clean with two kettlebells
- Bottoms up clean with press and one kettlebell
- Bottoms up clean with squat and one kettlebell

- Bottoms up clean with squat push press and one kettlebell
- Alternating bottoms up clean to bottoms up snatch with one kettlebell.

Exercise 100 Flipped clean with one kettlebell

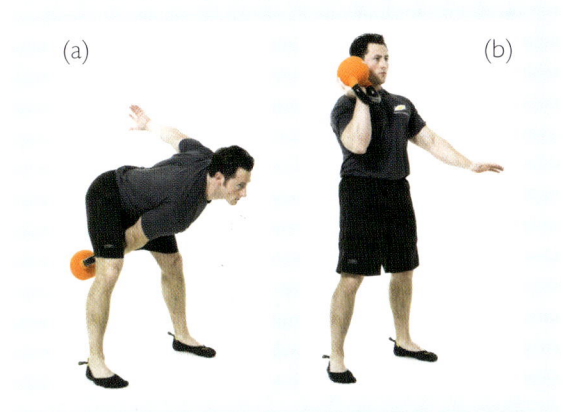

(a)   (b)

Just as with the snatch variation of this drill, the flipped clean is a great teaching drill to practise getting the kettlebell into the correct position for the standard clean. It is also a favourite juggling drill, even more so than the snatch variation, because the kettlebell is not going above the head.

Execution
- Swing the kettlebell as normal between the legs, extend the hips and pull upwards.
- As the kettlebell rises, release the handle so that it flips and catch the bell section in a cupped hand by the shoulder, with the forearm vertical and the handle down by the wrist.

- Pause briefly then push the kettlebell over, catch the handle on the descent, swing between the legs and repeat.

Exercise variations
Add any of the following progressions to this exercise for variation:

- Flipped grip press
- Flipped grip press to windmill
- Flipped grip press to overhead squat
- Flipped grip squat
- Flipped grip squat and press.

Exercise 101 Renegade row with two kettlebells

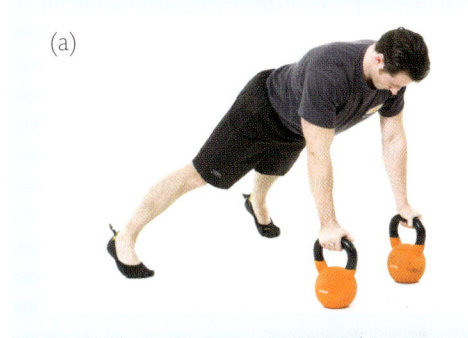

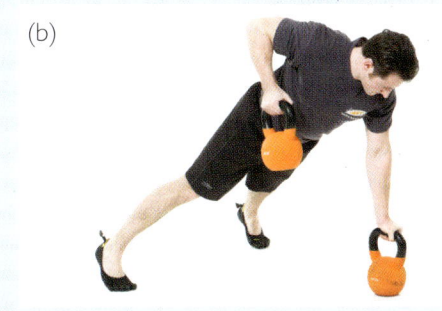

(a)

(b)

EXERCISE PROGRESSIONS

139

The renegade row is a great exercise that not only works the muscles of the back (the latissimus dorsi, erector spinae and rhomboids), but will also demand stability and control of the glutes, obliques and anterior core muscles. It is performed in a plank position with the aim to keep tension through the body in order to maintain a straight line from shoulder to hips in both stages of the movement.

Execution
- Start with the hands resting on the kettlebells directly under the shoulders.
- Keep the shoulders pulled down, away from the ears, and the core braced.
- Aim to keep level through the hips so that the weight is even into both knees, and press down strongly through one of the kettlebells. Support the lower body on the balls of the feet (keeping feet wider than the hips to make it easier to balance).
- Row one arm into the body as you push strongly into the resting kettlebell, while tightly contracting your glutes and abdominals to prevent a shifting through the hips.
- Lower the kettlebell back down to the floor, reset and repeat on the other side.
- Ensure that the kettlebells are stable enough to perform this drill; they should have a sufficient flat surface on the bottom otherwise the risk of injury will be much greater.

Key errors
- Rotation through the torso (see figure 10.2). This creates an excessive strain on the lower wrist and demonstrates a weak core. The challenge is to maintain a neutral alignment and counteract the rotational forces of lifting up one kettlebell.
- Shifting in the hips (see figure 10.3). This commonly exposes a weakness with the core and hip stabilisers and creates a faulty loading pattern.
- Rounding through the back or hunching in the shoulders. This presents in those with weak lower trapezius or rhomboids. As these muscles fatigue the upper trapezius will start to compensate, causing this deviation in the upper back.

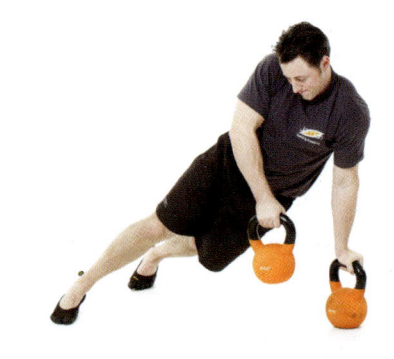

Figure 10.2 Rotation through the torso

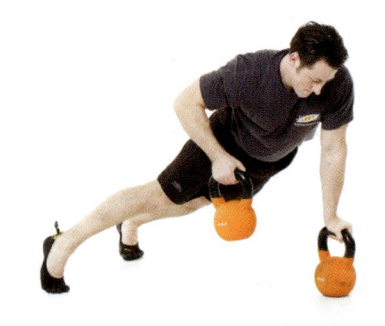

Figure 10.3 Shifting the hips

Exercise 102 Bent-over alternating row with two kettlebells

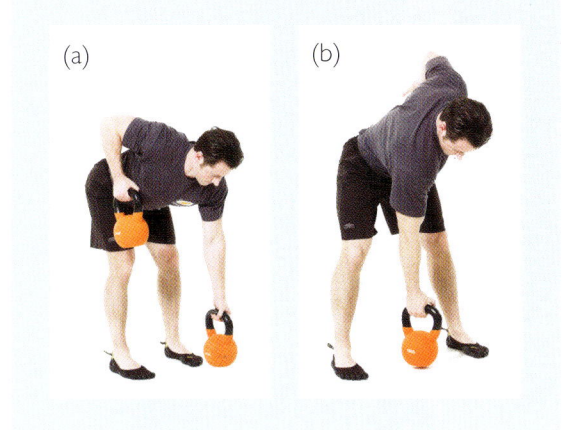

(a) (b)

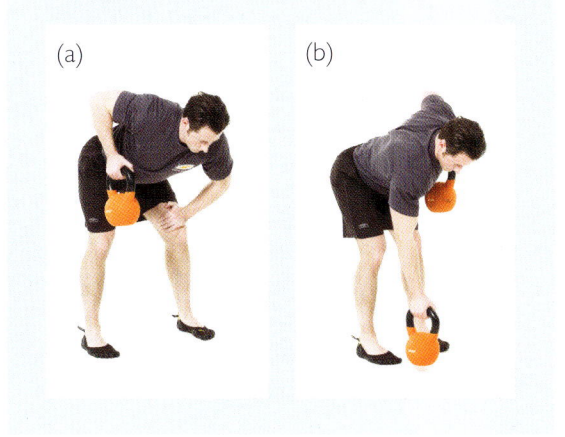

This exercise will predominantly work the latissimus dorsi, biceps and upper back muscles and is much easier than the renegade row.

Execution
- Stand in a parallel stance and lift up both kettlebells.
- Keeping the knees soft, bend over with the arms extended until the back position alters or just before the kettlebells reach the floor.
- Pull one kettlebell up to the side of the abdomen, keeping the spine neutral or flat.
- Slowly lower and at the same time pull the other kettlebell upwards.
- Alternate this motion, focusing on keeping the chest up throughout.

Exercise 103 Bent-over row with one kettlebell and arm support

(a) (b)

This variation is performed as a single sided exercise, which will be easier for beginners who have less core control.

Execution
- The hand that isn't holding the kettlebell is placed on the upper thigh of the front leg to aid stability and balance (a).
- Alternatively this single arm variation can also be performed without the arm support so that there is a unilateral loading effect (b), which further challenges the core stabilisers.

ROTATION PATTERN

Exercise 104 Seated rotations with one kettlebell

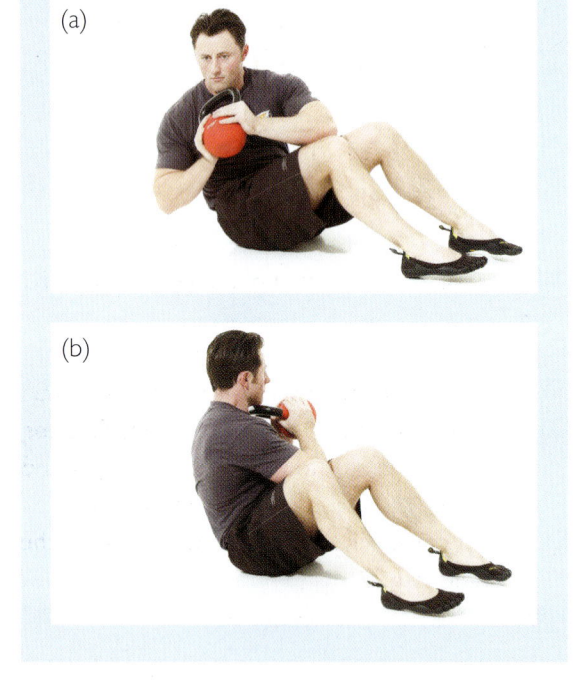

(a)

(b)

This exercise works the muscles of the core responsible for rotation and also recruits the stabilisers of the abdomen, lower back and the hip flexors. It is suitable for a range of individuals, but not those with a lower back weakness.

Execution
- Start seated with legs in front and slightly bent, feet on the floor.
- Keep the chest upright and brace the abdominals as you lean back, keeping the feet planted on the floor while holding the bell in both hands by the handle or crushing the bell.
- Keep the chest lifted as the kettlebell is rotated to one side of the body, then the other.
- For an additional challenge, perform this drill with the feet elevated off the ground.

Exercise 105 Standing crush grip rotation with one kettlebell

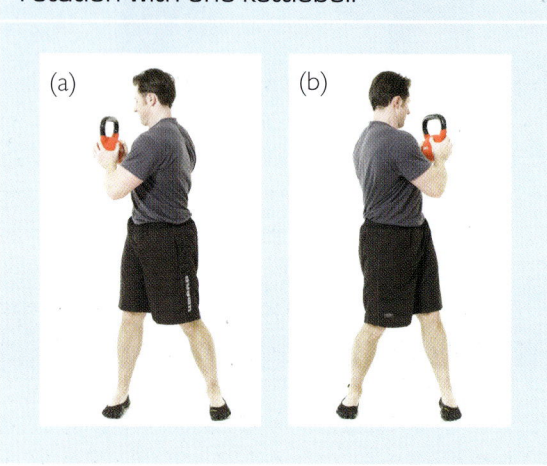

(a)   (b)

Execution
- Stand with feet shoulder width apart.
- Hold the bottom of the bell with both hands in a crush grip.
- Slowly rotate at the waist, first one way and then the other, keeping the bell at chest height.

Exercise variations
Variations of this exercise include:

- Standing with two heavy kettlebells in rack
- Standing with two kettlebells held overhead
- Kneeling or semi-kneeling position.

SMASH PATTERN

The smash pattern is a flexion movement of the torso. Examples of this human movement pattern in real life include throwing an object forward from overhead or slamming an axe straight downwards when chopping wood. It is not undertaken within life as frequently as lifting, and so should not be overtrained within an exercise programme.

CRUNCH EXERCISE

The crunch can be performed with a limited range of motion (purely spinal flexion), which will reduce potential stress on the structures of the back. For those with a history of back problems this may be a safer option.

There are strong proponents against doing any core training while in a supine position. For a number of sports, particularly the combative sports of MMA, wrestling and Jiu Jitsu, being strong on your back is very important for athletic success. It is therefore essential to train on the floor as well as to train standing.

Exercise 106 Crunch with one kettlebell

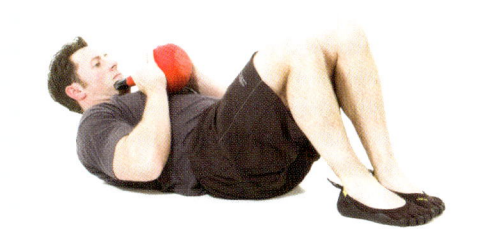

To get a full ROM, come up to a seated position.

Execution

- Hold the kettlebell by the horns or the actual bell, bring the chin to the chest and, focusing on a strong connection between the upper and lower body, come up to a seated position.
- Briefly pause, then lower slowly back to the start and repeat.

Exercise 107 Turkish get-up partial without hand support

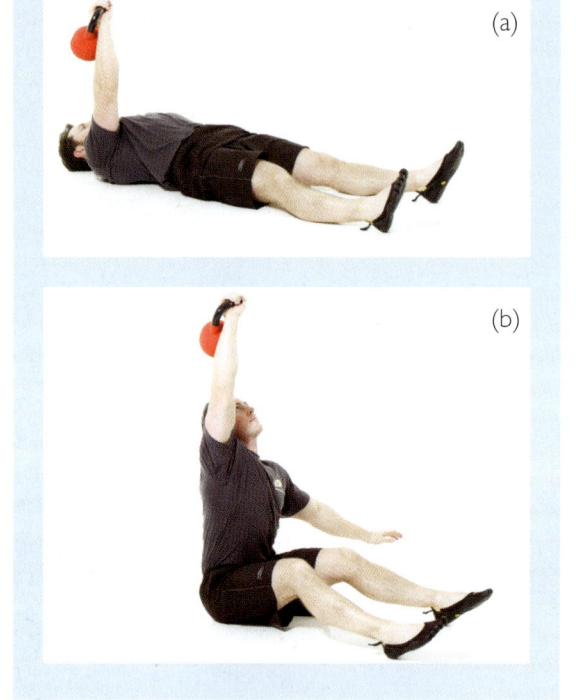

(a)

(b)

The Turkish get-up can be adapted to focus more on the anterior core and hip flexors used in the smash pattern.

Execution
- Perform the Turkish get-up as normal (see exercise 19, page 86), but only come up to the seated position, and don't use the other arm for support to push off the floor.
- Focus on a strong connection between the upper and lower body.
- Briefly hold then lower slowly back to the start position and repeat.

MOVING OR CARRYING LOAD PATTERN

The Turkish get-up is one of the best kettlebell exercises for this movement pattern – in this case moving a load from a supine to a standing position. A challenging variation of the traditional Turkish get-up is the squat variation. This requires greater mobility and stability through the shoulders and thoracic spine, as well as the ability to perform a deep overhead squat.

Exercise 108 Turkish get-up with squat and one kettlebell

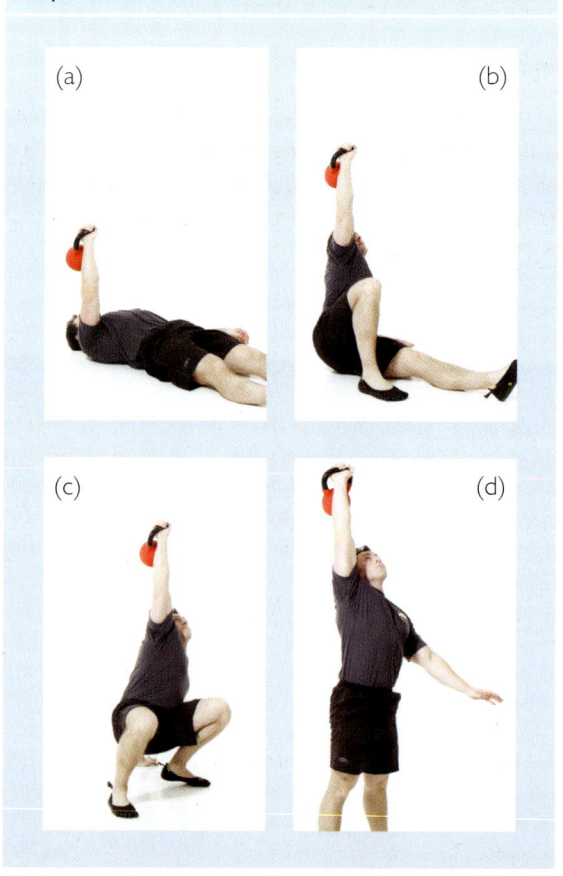

(a) (b)

(c) (d)

Execution
- Perform a Turkish get-up as normal (see exercise 19, page 86) until getting into the seated position.
- Lift the hips and straight leg off the ground, but instead of bringing it under the body to a kneeling position place the foot flat on the ground about shoulder width distance from the first foot (exercise 108c).
- Slide the supporting hand forward until all the weight is on the feet and then push up into a standing position.
- Squat down, place the hand down, slide the foot forward, sit down then return to the start position as normal and repeat.

Key errors
Be careful to watch out for the common error of lifting the heels off of the ground during the ascent or descent of the overhead squat phase (see figure 10.4) as this usually indicates restrictions in the foot or calf.

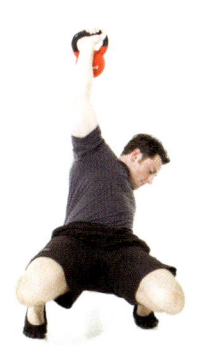

Figure 10.4 Lifting the heels of the ground

Exercise 109 Get up anyhow with two kettlebells

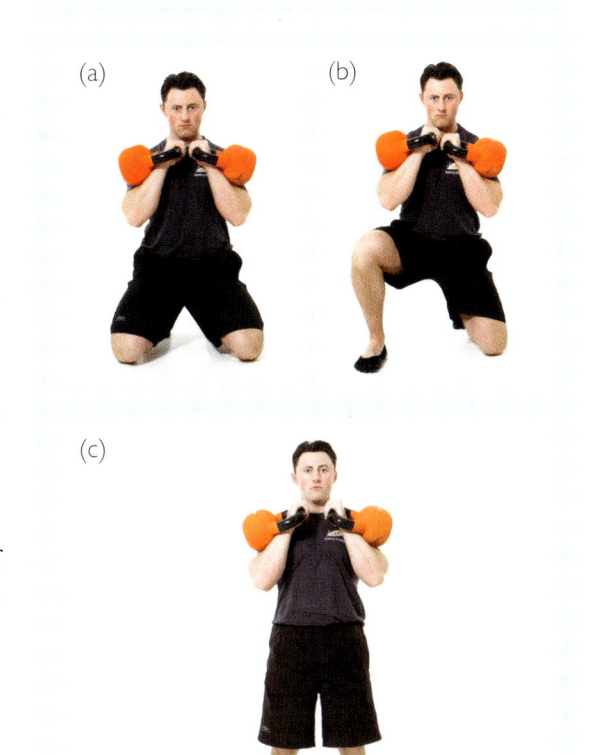

The get up anyhow is along the same lines as the two hands anyhow (exercise 89, page 132), but instead of trying to lift both kettlebells above the head with any technique available, the idea is to go from a supine or seated position to a standing position holding either one kettlebell in both hands or two kettlebells in two hands.

This type of drill is great when an individual is normally reliant upon their hands to assist them, for example, it is a great drill for MMA fighters who must get off the floor while holding an opponent away with their arms.

Execution
- As can be seen in the images shown, Marc has gone from a seated position into a kneeling position and then to standing with two kettlebells in the rack position.
- Not being able to use the hands for balance or to push off the floor means that the core and hip stabilisers have to work harder.

Exercise 110 Farmer's walk with two kettlebells

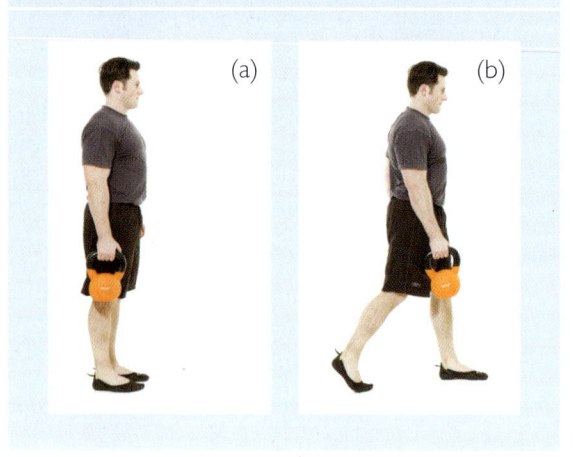

(a) (b)

The farmer's walk is one of the best exercises for improving grip strength and endurance as well and upper back endurance and even hip, core and ankle stability.

Execution
- Deadlift the kettlebells up from the floor.
- Hold a heavy kettlebell in either hand and walk for a set distance, or time, in a figure of eight pattern.

Exercise variations
There are several variations of this exercise, which should also be tried:

- Farmer's walk with two kettlebells in one hand (really tough on the grip)
- Farmer's walk with one kettlebell (further loads the lateral core and can be performed with the other hand on top of the head)
- Farmer's walk with two kettlebells and towel grip (varies the stress on the hand and grip muscles).

Exercise 111 Walk with one kettlebell held overhead

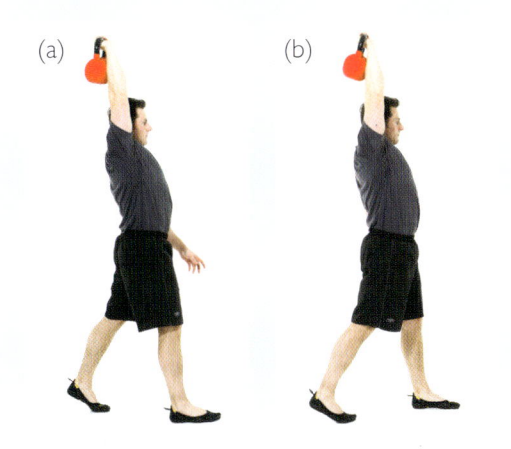

(a)　(b)

Many of the moving load drills are rarely seen in a standard gym environment, but exercises like the walk with bell held overhead really challenge the core and shoulder stabilisers.

Execution
- Lift the kettlebell up to a position above the head in whatever technique is easiest – clean and jerk/press, snatch, etc.
- Make sure the kettlebell is nice and heavy and slowly walk for a set distance or time.

Exercise variations
This exercise can also be performed with two kettlebells, one in each hand, or for less shoulder involvement use two kettlebells held in the rack position.

Exercise 112 Supine shuffle with one kettlebell held above the head

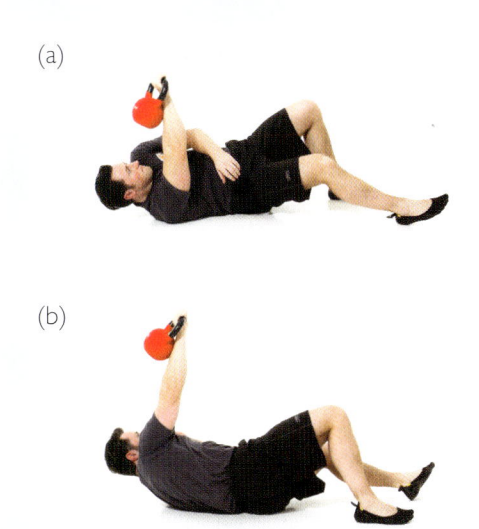

(a)

(b)

Execution
- Lie on the floor in a supine position.
- Hold a single kettlebell above the body, and use the core and legs to move along the floor.
- Avoid using the other arm, which can also hold another kettlebell for an additional challenge, and make sure that you are always watching the kettlebell and keeping it under control.

EXERCISE PROGRESSIONS

GAIT AND LOCOMOTION

The gait and locomotion movement pattern includes walking, running, crawling and swimming. Obviously this movement pattern is performed without any external load (otherwise it comes under the moving-carrying load pattern), and thus for kettlebell training does not have exercises listed under it.

SUPPLEMENTARY DRILLS

Any drills that do not easily fit into one of the before mentioned human movement patterns are classed as supplementary exercises. These should be viewed as potentially beneficial in strengthening any weak areas involved in the press, pull or any other movement pattern. Examples of supplementary exercises include:

- hammer curls with one kettlebell
- plank on two kettlebells with knee raise

Exercise 113 Hammer curls with one kettlebell

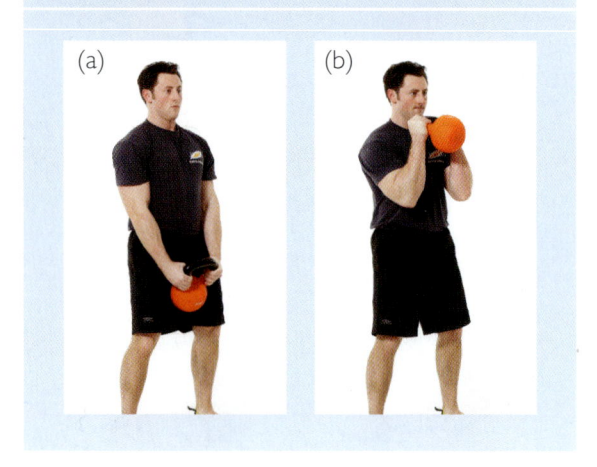

Execution
- Hold the kettlebell by the horns in a semi-supinated position.
- Curl the kettlebell up, gripping the horns tightly to ensure it doesn't fall.
- For a variation, feed a towel through each kettlebell handle and hold the towels with a semi-supinated grip to curl up the kettlebell.

Exercise 114 Plank on two kettlebells with knee raise

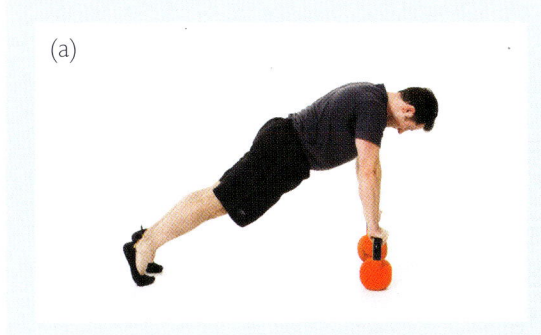

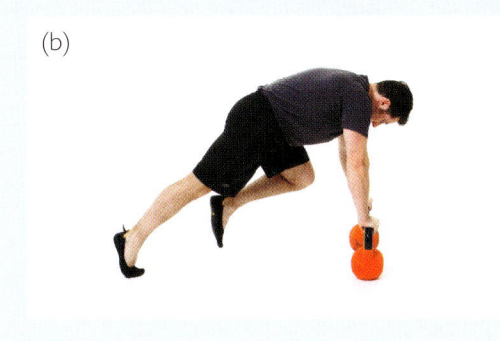

(a)

(b)

This is a variation of the standard plank drill, but is harder on the shoulder and scapula stabilisers.

Execution
- Place two kettlebells about shoulder width apart.
- With arms extended, place weight onto the bells and extend the legs behind into a full plank position.
- Keeping the hips and torso still, lift one knee up towards the chest.
- Push back to the original position and repeat on both sides.

There are probably many other drills or variations that can be used with kettlebells. Good trainers and instructors will experiment with equipment to find new ways of getting results with their clients.

3

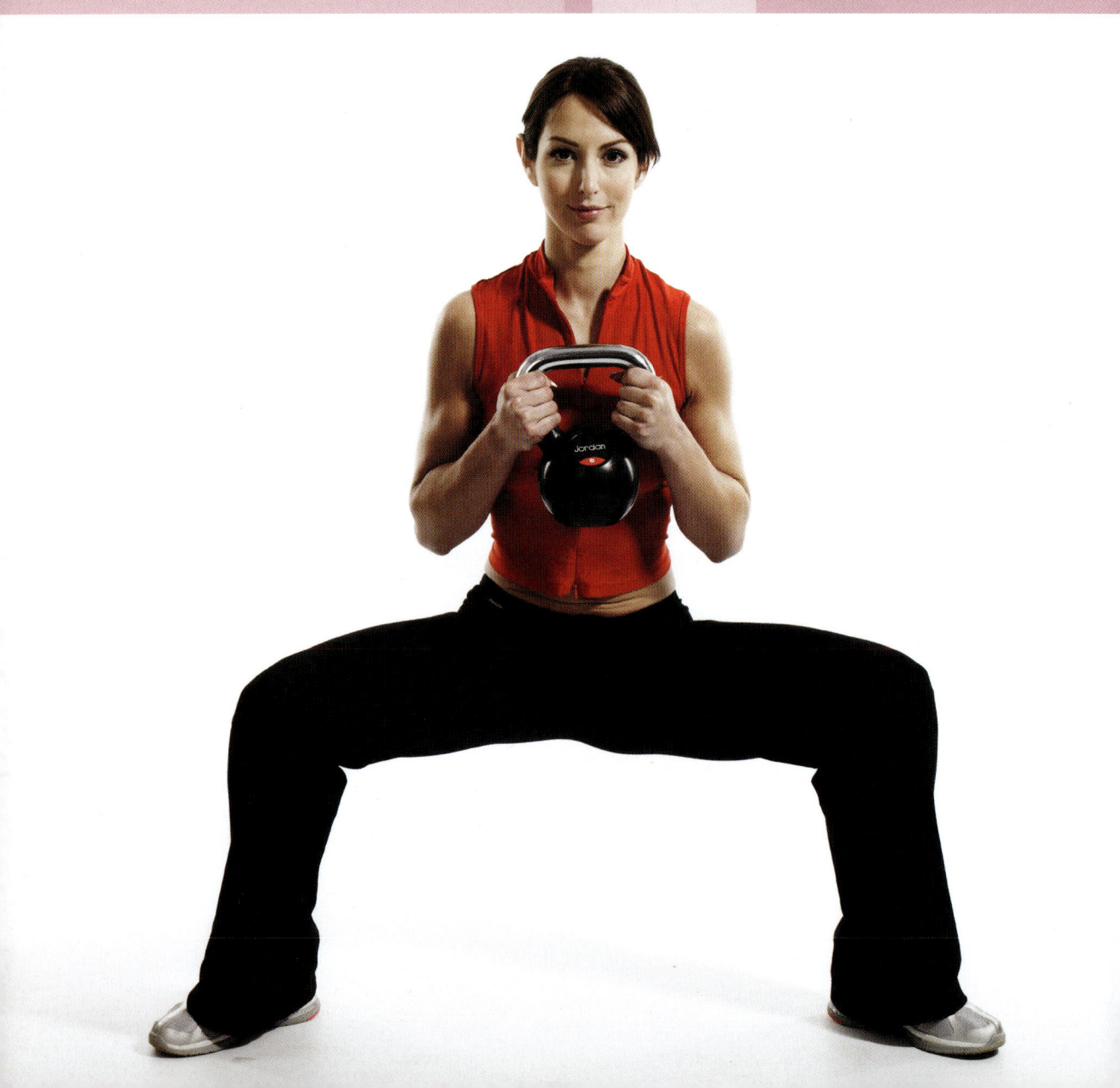

PART THREE

TRAINING RECOMMENDATIONS

TRAINING PARAMETERS AND APPLICATION

11

TRAINING PRINCIPLES

All training programmes should adhere to the key principles of training:

- Adaptation
- Overload
- Specificity
- Reversibility
- Acclimatisation
- Periodisation

ADAPTATION

Adaptation is any anatomical or physiological change in the body caused by a stimulus or stressor. Improvements in VO_2max, decreased body fat percentage, increased absolute strength on the back squat, increased bone density and improved insulin sensitivity are all examples of how the body may change and alter to the particular stresses it is exposed to in order to survive and flourish in this new and changing environment.

OVERLOAD

Overload is the stimulus or stressor, which must be above a minimum threshold in order to cause an adaptation. Whatever the adaptation sought, the overload must be above a certain threshold in order to elicit this change (to stimulate the body to adapt), while not becoming an excessive overload. Insufficient overload will not cause an adaptation, while excessive overload will be too stressful to the body and therefore may also impede the desired change. The idea is to pitch the overload between these two levels (in relation to intensity, density or volume).

Plateau busters

Periods of short-term overreaching sessions or training are commonly called plateau busters. They are designed to 'shock' the body into adapting to change. It may seem like excessive overload in the short term, but in the long term it can cause improved adaptations, as long as it is carefully applied so as not to cause the body to go into an overtraining state.

SPECIFICITY

Specificity means that the adaptation will be specialised and exact in response to the particular overload. There will always be a specificity buffer when applying overload, and it doesn't have to be exactly the same as the activity you are looking to improve, but it should be similar in relation to:

- muscles activated;
- motor units recruited;
- tempo and time-under-tension (TUT);
- energy systems worked;
- type of muscle contraction;
- joints used;
- force vector (the angle or direction that the load is moved – for example, the press pattern could be vertical upwards, vertical downwards, horizontal, diagonal upwards, diagonal downwards);
- movement pattern;
- load;
- intensity; and
- recovery period between bouts of activity.

Analysing the activity and then choosing the correct training variables will help accomplish similarities, but supplementary drills and cross-training can also have a beneficial outcome in relation to performance, despite the activity not being exactly the same. For example, isolated seated leg curls on a fixed path machine can help to improve hamstring strength, correct medial to lateral head imbalances, balance quad to hamstring strength ratios and improve knee stability, which when applied with appropriate squat pattern exercises can help to improve the functional capabilities of sprinting, jumping and throwing.

REVERSIBILITY

Reversibility states that no adaptation is permanent; the overload must be maintained, varied or increased or the changes will eventually diminish to pre-training levels. Training variables must be manipulated and stress continued to be applied to continue adaptations and prevent adaptations being lost. Periodisation will help to maintain adaptations from previous phases of training while new adaptations are being sought.

ACCLIMATISATION

Acclimatisation states that the body will gradually adapt to a particular stimulus or stressor, diminishing its effects and benefits. Some individuals will acclimatise very quickly, while others will continue to benefit and adapt to similar stresses (the same session) applied over longer periods of time.

Clients gifted with high proportions of fast twitch fibres will usually adapt quicker to a stimulus, and thus will need to vary the session more frequently, while most clients will usually be able to follow the same session (with small micro-changes) five to seven times before needing significant variation. Manipulating the training variables at an appropriate time, alongside correct recovery periods between sessions and phases of training, and the input of 'shock training' will all help to prevent or limit plateauing of improvements or adaptations.

PERIODISATION

Periodisation states that in order to prevent acclimatisation the training overload should be progressively manipulated and integrated with recovery periods to more effectively elicit the adaptations of training. Twelve-week work cycles, broken down into smaller phases and then into individual sessions, work very well for most individuals, with one to two weeks of recovery between the cycles. Frequency of sessions, multiple sessions per day and tolerance to intensity and volume will greatly depend on the individual and their training experience.

HUMAN MOVEMENT PATTERNS

As we discovered in chapter 3, the foundation human movement patterns are:

- Squat
- Lift
- Pull
- Press
- Rotate
- Smash
- Moving or carrying load
- Gait and locomotion.

These movement patterns should be an integral part of every strength and conditioning programme, whether it is the programme of an athlete or a non-athlete. Every individual should be evaluated in their efficiency to demonstrate each of these movement patterns, as well as those movement patterns that may be more specific to the client's vocation or sport.

SUPPLEMENTARY MOVEMENTS OR EXERCISES

Any movements or exercises that don't fit into any of the human movement patterns listed above can be grouped under this category. Exercises such as the leg extension, leg curl or shoulder external rotation can have a positive influence on the squat, lift and press patterns respectively and could therefore be included within a training programme focused on these areas. Just like dietary supplements, these exercises should complement the basic exercises for movement patterns and should not replace them.

Some exercises will be classified as a combination of movement patterns, for example:

- The clean is a combination of a lift and pull (vertical upwards) pattern. In a (swing) clean, the lift pattern dominates as the pull with the upper body is less significant, being more of a redirection of the force generated by the swing (lift) phase.
- The hang dead clean recruits more of a pull (vertical upwards) pattern, as there is no pre-loading phase for the posterior chain (lifting muscles) and they will therefore be able to contribute less energy to bringing the kettlebell up to the rack position.

Examples of supplementary exercises include:

- Towel bicep curl with one kettlebell (a supplementary exercise for the pull pattern).
- Side plank (a supplementary exercise for the press and lift patterns).

CATEGORISATION OF KETTLEBELL EXERCISES

Table 11.1 shows a selection of kettlebell exercises and variations demonstrated in this book that fit into the major movement patterns. These patterns allow for the full spectrum of human movements to be improved within the training programme.

Table 11.1 Example kettlebell exercises grouped by human movement patterns

Movement pattern	Sub-group	Example kettlebell exercise
Squat	Parallel stance	Kettlebell front squat (exercise 17, page 79)
	Split stance	Kettlebell overhead split squat (variation of exercise 72, page 121)
	Single leg stance	Kettlebell pistol squat (exercise 68, page 118)
	Dynamic (lunge)	Kettlebell walking lunge (variation of exercise 73, page 122)
Lift	Slow	Kettlebell good morning (exercise 35, page 99)
	Dynamic	Kettlebell swing (exercise 5, page 57)
Pull	Vertical upwards	Kettlebell high pull (exercise 10, page 68)
	Horizontal	Kettlebell bent-over row (exercise 103, page 141)
	Vertical downwards	Bodyweight pull-up*
Press	Vertical upwards	Kettlebell overhead press (exercise 18, page 82)
	Horizontal	Kettlebell bridge press (exercise 91, page 133)
	Vertical downwards	Bodyweight dips*
Rotate	Horizontal	Kettlebell seated rotations (exercise 104, page 142)
	Diagonal upwards	Kettlebell diagonal dead snatch (exercise 44, page 106)
	Diagonal downwards	Cable woodchop*
Smash	Supine	Supine crunch holding a kettlebell (exercise 106, page 143)
	Standing	Standing medicine ball throw forwards
Moving or carrying load	From supine	Kettlebell Turkish get-up (exercise 19, page 86)
	In the hands	Kettlebell farmer's walk (exercise 110, page 146)
Gait and locomotion	Always undertaken unloaded	

* Like many functional tools, the kettlebell does not adequately cover all possible movement patterns. These exercises are examples of those that complement kettlebell training.

TRAINING RECOMMENDATIONS

INTENSITY

Intensity is a term commonly used in the fitness industry to describe how hard a session is, but this definition is too watery and actually incorrect. When intensity is described in relation to lifting weights it refers to how close to 1 repetition maximum (RM) or what percentage of 1RM is being lifted. No matter what the desired training effect, the individual must look to go to failure in order to elicit that effect. Lifting a weight in eight repetitions that is so light it could be lifted 20 times has limited benefit, as it won't overload the body sufficiently to cause any adaptations. Beginners have a low threshold for improvements in strength, and thus will respond to a low intensity with higher repetitions.

> **Repetition maximum (RM)**
> RM infers that the maximum weight is lifted for the number given, i.e. 1RM means the maximum weight for one repetition, while a 6–8RM means that the chosen weight should cause the individual to go to concentric failure between the sixth and eighth repetition

As we have discussed, kettlebell training is designed to work the strength-endurance range of the strength spectrum, rather than maximal strength. Usually, when choosing to improve maximal strength, a more stable, heavier tool is used, such as a barbell. For example, a barbell deadlift and a kettlebell swing both improve the posterior chain muscles. The barbell deadlift may be trained for 6–8 repetitions at 140kg. Could a 140kg kettlebell be swung for 8 reps? Of course not. Even the heaviest kettlebells at 40kg are very light in comparison with barbell loads. These lighter tools are therefore better utilised for sustained, longer sets, with more repetitions, performed ballistically and with comparatively lower loads.

Choosing the right load

In terms of kettlebells loads, the weight of the kettlebell will vary depending on the exercise being performed. Usually the heaviest loads can be used with the two hand swing and the clean, as the two hand swing is the most stable of the dynamic drills because it is held with both hands, and the clean because it only needs to be lifted to about hip height and incorporates the lifting and pulling muscles. The one hand swing and the one hand snatch usually demand a slightly lighter bell, because the one hand swing will be more imbalanced than the two hand, and because the snatch has to travel further (higher) than the clean. The slower tempo strength exercises, such as the one hand press and Turkish get-up, require the lightest kettlebells because of the lack of momentum and elastic energy needed to perform these exercises and the higher degree of stabiliser fatigue involved in those drills.

For certain exercises, such as the snatch and the clean, using too light a load can make it difficult to learn the correct technique and motor activation. Too light a kettlebell when performing a snatch commonly makes it difficult to correctly learn the extend-pull-punch timing, and may well cause the bell to bang on the forearm.

REPETITIONS

The selection of an appropriate repetition range is probably the most important training variable in resistance training programming. The repetition range will influence other training variables such as the tempo, sets, rest and, of course, the intensity. Intensity and repetition range are intrinsically linked and inversely proportional; as the repetition range decreases, the intensity increases.

With any complex multiple-joint exercises, excessive repetitions and fatigue may bring about undesirable motor learning and technical changes (Poliquin, 2004). This is the case when learning and training with kettlebells. Although not as proprioceptively challenging as the barbell snatch or clean, it will still be better to perform multiple sets of lower repetitions when learning in order to ensure optimal motor programming. As clients get more acclimatised to the drills, the number of repetitions can be increased to develop a higher level of work capacity.

Time-under-tension (TUT) and repetitions

For certain cyclical drills, such as the swings, it may be better to use TUT as the focal parameter rather than repetitions, because of the fast tempo of each repetition. A client may only complete 15 seconds of work for a 10-repetition set. If the client is after more strength-endurance, they should look for a time-under-tension range of 50–120 seconds.

We should also consider TUT at the other end of the scale, i.e. in those exercises with a slow tempo for each repetition. For certain exercises such as a Turkish get-up, excessive repetitions are counterproductive since stabilising muscles, such as the deltoids and trapezius, fatigue quickly and cause changes in technique. To prevent this, most strength coaches keep the repetitions on the low side, up to 4–8, with sets lasting 20-40 seconds.

TEMPO

Tempo can be defined as the speed of movement for an exercise. Many strength coaches will say that tempo is one of the training variables, if not *the* training variable, that is most neglected for variation within a periodised programme (King, 2000; Poliquin, 2004). In fact, variation in the tempo may be critical for prolonged strength development (Bührle and Schmidtbleicher, 1981), particularly for elite athletes in power sports.

Some trainers may describe the desired tempo for their selected exercise in very basic terms (slow, moderate, fast...), but this is simply insufficient for a modern professional in the health and fitness industry. There are several different methods for indicating the tempo to be trained to the client, and the following is the most comprehensive.

Example exercise focused on varying tempo

Exercise	Sets	Reps	Tempo	Rest period (s)
Kettlebell front squat	3	6–8	4.1.1.0.	120

The four-digit code shown in the tempo column is used to describe the tempo for the different phases of a resistance exercise: eccentric, isometric, concentric, isometric. Using the example of the front squat, a client would undertake the following tempo:

- Eccentric phase (the controlling phase from the standing position to the bottom position): 4 seconds
- Isometric phase (the pause in the bottom position): 1 second
- Concentric phase (the exerting phase from the bottom position to the standing position): 1 second
- Isometric phase (the pause in the standing position): 0 seconds.

This gives you the four-digit code: 4.1.1.0. Using this example, each repetition takes a total of 6 seconds to complete, which becomes very important when calculating the TUT for a set. If a trainer wishes to have their client undertake a phase as fast as possible (normally during the concentric phase), then an 'X' can be used, i.e. the tempo for the front squat with a fast concentric phase is written as 4.1.X.0.

This system can cause some trainers or clients to get confused with most pulling exercises, since they tend to begin with the concentric phase first.

The numerical system does not change for each exercise, since this causes more confusion. No matter whether the exercise is executed with a concentric or eccentric phase first, it is always written in the order of eccentric, isometric, concentric, isometric.

The speed of the movement determines a number of factors, including the amount of tension developed, the use of mechanical energy (such as the stretch-shortening cycle), and the load (King, 2000). This obviously has implications for the outcome of the training effect, for example, the mechanical properties of the stretch-shortening cycle elicit neurological adaptations, while increasing muscular tension can promote morphological changes (i.e. hypertrophy, the increase of muscle cells).

Tempo and time-under-tension

The term 'time-under-tension' has been used for decades and describes how long a muscle or group of muscles is under contractile stress. TUT is calculated by multiplying the number of repetitions by the tempo or total time for each repetition. For example, if 6 reps of the front squat were performed at a tempo of 4.1.1.0, then the total TUT for that set would be 6 x 6 seconds, or 36 seconds. The following table describes the training effect elicited from different times under tension (adapted from King, 2000):

Table 11.2 Training effects elicited from varying TUT

TUT	Dominanet training effect
1–20 seconds	Speed strength/maximal strength
20–40 seconds	Functional strength
40–70 seconds	Hypertrophy
50–120 seconds	Strength endurance

As previously mentioned, the general goal of using the kettlebell is to improve strength-endurance. Therefore, sets should ideally last for at least 50 seconds. For many individuals, undertaking repeated bouts of 20–30 seconds might be preferable, with 10–15 seconds rest periods in between. This allows them to maintain a high quality of technique, whereas prolonged sets can sometimes cause the technique to falter. Although small, the 10–15 second rest periods help to maintain this quality.

Selection of the mid-isometric tempo will vary depending on the desired training effect. If more muscular tension is desired for hypertrophying effects, then the isometric pause should be increased to reduce the effect of the stretch-shortening cycle. Research shows that this should be up to 4 seconds to eliminate the elastic energy from the eccentric phase (Wilson et al., 1991). For strength training this period should be between 0–2 seconds and for power training it should be 0 seconds, i.e. in exercises such as the swing, clean and snatch.

For fast (signified by an 'X') tempos, it is critical that a basic threshold of strength is achieved prior to commencement of explosive strength regimes. Since the swings, cleans and snatches are all performed at a maximal velocity, they should always be preceded with slower tempo exercises to strengthen the posterior chain, such as Romanian deadlifts (RDLs).

An example of how to write the optimal tempo for certain ballistic and slower drills are given on the following page:

Table 11.3 Example exercises for optimal tempo

Exercise and tempo	Breakdown of tempo
Front squat 3.1.1.1.	3 seconds on the way down
	1 second pause at the bottom
	1 second on the way up
	1 second hold in an upright position
Two hand swing X.0.X.0.	X – the bell is swung between the legs at quite a fast velocity
	0 seconds for pause at bottom
	X – the bell is projected upwards as fast as possible
	0 seconds for pause at top
One hand snatch X.0.X.2	X – the bell is swung between the legs at quite a fast velocity
	0 seconds for pause at bottom
	X – the bell is projected upwards as fast as possible
	2 second hold once the bell has reached the top position before dropping into the next rep

SETS AND VOLUME

The manipulation of the number of sets when programming is a key parameter in the pursuit of strength. The use of multiple sets leads to higher and quicker gains in strength, and for each training effect there is an optimal and upper limit to the number of sets required.

For strength endurance, I recommend two to four sets per exercise, while hypertrophy requires four to eight sets per exercise. Use more sets to elicit gains in size and/or for functional and relative strength. Hypertrophy gains are triggered by the greater volume causing increases in testosterone and growth hormone (Kraemer et al., 1990). If a programme has only a few specific exercises, then more sets should be completed to focus strength in particular planes or for particular movement patterns. Use less sets with exercises with larger repetition ranges, longer TUT or in sessions with more exercises.

Elite kettlebell competitors perform hundreds of repetitions over multiple sets to grove the motor patterns for the snatch, jerk and clean, since these are the exercises they need to focus on for their sport. All other drills are supplementary to their performance in these exercises.

REST PERIODS

The key to selecting the appropriate rest period is to focus on which training goal you are targeting. The higher the intensity and the lower the repetition range, the longer the rest periods. For strength-endurance it is recommended to use a rest period of 10–90 seconds between sets. Selection of the rest period will vary depending on the exercise. Exercises that have a longer range of motion, that recruit more muscle mass or are neurologically more demanding will require longer rest periods for adequate recovery. Intra-set rest periods of 10–20 seconds may well help maintain a high quality of technique during a set, but may also favour the recruitment of the higher threshold motor units.

The rest interval can be manipulated to affect the hormonal response. Keeping the rest intervals shorter will increase production of testosterone (Fry et al., 1994) and growth hormone (Kraemer et al., 1990). Pairing antagonistic (opposing) muscle groups, such as push-pull muscles in the upper body or upper-lower body pairs, can allow for shorter rest periods and a larger volume of work for the session.

For training in the lactate power range of 20–40 seconds TUT, you should follow with a rest period of 120–180 seconds. For lactate capacity training of 40–70 seconds TUT, you would have a rest period of 90–120 seconds. It is common to super-set or semi-super-set compatible kettlebell or non-kettlebell exercises to maximise work density within a session.

Trainers should try to avoid overloading the same myofascial meridians (or groups of muscles), such as the superficial back line and functional back line with similar exercises. For example, the snatch (let's refer to this as A1) and the swing (A2). These exercises both work the posterior chain muscles resulting in excessive local muscular fatigue for beginners.

Order

Because many kettlebell exercises are dynamic and are complex multi-joint exercises, they should be undertaken towards the beginning of the session, after a warm-up and prior to fatiguing assistant strength exercises performed at slow tempos. When exercises are written as part of a programme, the following letter-number system is used:

Example 1

Order	Exercise	Reps/rest	Sets
A1	Exercise 1	10 reps /30s	3 sets
A2	Exercise 2	10 reps /30s	3 sets

So, in this example, exercise 1 is super-setted with exercise 2. Exercise 1 is performed for 10 reps, then 30 seconds' rest, then exercise 2 is performed for 10 reps then 30 seconds' rest, and then back to exercise 1. Each exercise is performed for three sets in total.

Example 2

Order	Exercise	Reps/rest	Sets
A1	Exercise 1	10 reps 30s	3 sets
B1	Exercise 2	10 reps 30s	3 sets

In this example, exercise 1 is performed for 10 reps, then 30 seconds' rest, and then it is performed again. This continues until all three sets have been completed, before moving on to exercise 2.

EXAMPLE TRAINING SESSIONS 12

BEGINNER SESSIONS
Here are several examples of kettlebell sessions designed for beginners and using the foundation exercises demonstrated in chapter 9.

Beginner session 1 using foundation exercises

Warm-up drills: 10 minutes

Order	Exercise	TUT (s)	Tempo	Rest (s)	Sets	Notes
A1	Swing left hand	20	X.0.X.1.	10	2	Rest 120 seconds and repeat x 3
A2	Swing right hand	20	X.0.X.1.	10	2	
B1	Squat left hand	20	3.1.X.1.	10	2	Rest 120 seconds and repeat x 3
B2	Squat right hand	20	3.1.X.1.	10	2	
C1	Press left hand	20	3.0.1.1	10	2	Rest 120 seconds and repeat x 3
C2	Press right hand	20	3.0.1.1	10	2	

Weekly beginner programme 1

Day	Session
Monday	Session 1
Tuesday	Weights session to include pull-ups, rotation and Turkish get-ups
Wednesday	Rest
Thursday	Session 1
Friday	Weights session to include pull-ups, rotation and Turkish get-ups
Saturday	Rest
Sunday	Rest

Beginner session 2 using more drills

Warm-up drills	10 minutes					

Order	Exercise	TUT (s)/RM	Tempo	Rest (s)	Sets	Notes
A1	Two hand swings	20s	X.0.X.1.	10	4	
A2	Windmill	30s	3.1.1.1.	30	4	
B1	Pull-ups	8RM	3.1.X.0.	45	3	Alternate Windmill sides between each set of swings
B2	Front squats	40s	3.1.X.0.	45	3	
C1	Press-ups closed grip	10RM	3.1.1.1	15	3	
C2	Low cable seated row	12RM	3.1.1.1	45	3	

Weekly beginner programme 2

Day	Session
Monday	Session 2
Tuesday	Sprint interval session
Wednesday	Rest
Thursday	Session 2
Friday	Swim interval session
Saturday	Session 2
Sunday	Rest

INTERMEDIATE SESSIONS

Follow these example session plans if you have progressed beyond beginner level. The first intermediate session is based on the Tabata Protocol (20 second high intensity, 10 seconds rest, repeat for 8 sets).

Intermediate session 1 using Tabata Protocol

Warm-up drills: 10 minutes

Order	Exercise	TUT (s)/RM	Tempo	Rest (s)	Sets	Notes
A1	Clean left hand side	20	X.0.X.1.	10	4–5	
A2	Clean right hand side	20	X.0.X.1.	10	4–5	
A3	Swing left hand side	20	X.0.X.0.	10	4–5	
A4	Swing right hand side	20	X.0.X.0.	10	4–5	Perform exercises A1 to A8. Rest for 180 seconds then repeat for a total of 4–5 times.
A5	Squat left hand side	20	2.0.X.0.	10	4–5	
A6	Press left hand side	20	2.0.X.0.	10	4–5	
A7	Squat right hand side	20	2.0.X.0.	10	4–5	
A8	Press right hand side	20	2.0.X.0.	180	4–5	

For the following session you should use a suitable suspension system such as a Milo Kit or TRX.

Intermediate session 2 using suspension system

Warm-up drills	10 minutes					

Order	Exercise	TUT (s)/RM	Tempo	Rest (s)	Sets	Notes
A1	Dead snatch left hand side	20	0.1.X.1.	10	4–5	
A2	Dead snatch right hand side	20	0.1.X.1.	10	4–5	Perform exercises A1 to A8. Rest for 120 seconds then repeat for a total of 4–5 times.
A3	Suspension system rows	20	2.1.X.1.	10	4–5	
A4	Squat push press	20	1.0.X.0.	10	4–5	
A5	Suspension system jack knife	20	2.0.X.0.	10	4–5	
A6	Swing left hand side	20	X.0.X.0.	10	4–5	
A7	Swing right hand side	20	X.0.X.0.	10	4–5	
A8	Suspension system chest press	20	2.0.X.1.	120	4–5	

This third intermediate session follows a 6-12-25 Protocol, as shown in the table, with lift and squat patterns. Three exercises are put together, with 6RM for the first exercise, 12RM on the second exercise and 25RM for the third exercise.

Intermediate session 3 using 6–12–25 Protocol

Warm-up drills	10 minutes					

Order	Exercise	TUT (s)/RM	Tempo	Rest (s)	Sets	Notes
A1	Barbell deadlift	6RM	3.1.X.1.	10	5	These three will overload the lift pattern muscles
A2	Glute-ham raise	12RM	3.1.X.1.	10	5	
A3	Hand to hand swing	25RM	X.0.X.0.	180	5	
B1	Barbell front squat	6RM	3.1.X.1.	10	5	These three will overload the squat pattern muscles
B2	Kettlebell racked lunges	12RM	1.0.X.1.	10	5	
B3	Seated Leg extension	25RM	2.1.1.1.	180	5	

Intermediate session 4 focuses on whole body resistance.

Intermediate session 4 using whole body resistance

| Warm-up drills | 10 minutes | | | | | |

Order	Exercise	TUT (s)/RM	Tempo	Rest (s)	Sets	Notes
A1	Snatch lift	45	X.1.X.1.	60	5	
A2	Windmill left	45	3.1.1.1.	60	5	
A3	Snatch right	45	X.0.X.1.	60	5	
A4	Windmill right	45	3.1.1.1.	60	5	
A5	Two hand jerks with two kettlebells	45	X.0.X.1.	60	5	

ADVANCED SESSIONS

Follow these example session plans if you have progressed beyond intermediate level. The first intermediate session combines both the barbell and the kettlebell.

Advanced session 1 using kettlebell-barbell combination

| Warm-up drills | 10 minutes | | | | | |

Order	Exercise	TUT (s)/RM	Tempo	Rest (s)	Sets	Notes
A1	Barbell snatch	3RM	0.1.X.1.	10	4	
A2	Kettlebell snatch*	60	X.0.X.1.	180	4	
B1	Barbell clean	5RM	0.1.X.1.	10	4	
B2	Kettlebell clean with two bells	60	X.0.X.1.	180	4	*Alternate sides every 2 reps
C1	Barbell power jerk	4RM	X.0.X.1.	10	4	
C2	Kettlebell power jerk with two bells	60	X.0.X.1.	180	4	

This session will help you to prepare for competitions.

Advanced session 2 kettlebell competition practice						
Warm-up drills	10 minutes					
Order	Exercise	TUT (s)/RM	Tempo	Rest (s)	Sets	Notes
A1	Snatch left hand	60	X.0.X.2.	30	4	
B1	Snatch right hand	60	X.0.X.2.	30	4	
C1	Two hand jerk	60	X.0.X.1.	30	8	

Build up the number of sets to 5 for the snatch and 10 for the jerk over a period of time, and decrease the rest period from 30 seconds. Use any accessory drills in additional to develop strength endurance or muscular balance.

COMPETITIVE KETTLEBELL LIFTING

13

There are a number of regional, national and international governing bodies that promote the sport of kettlebell lifting. The largest of these and the most prominent are the World Kettlebell Club (WKC), the International Union of Kettlebell Lifting (IUKL) and the IGSF (International Girya Sport Federation).

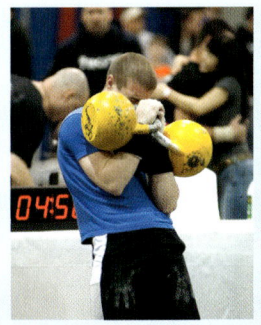

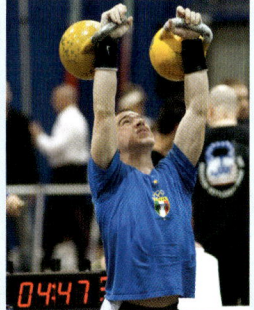

Figure 13.1 Girevoy Rack in competition (left), Girevoy Jerk in competition (right).

There are two disciplines in kettlebell competitions; the biathlon and the long cycle. The biathlon is actually made up of two events – the jerk (two hand for males, one hand for females) and the snatch (one hand). The long cycle is a two hand clean and jerk. The bell weights used in competitions are 12, 16, 24, and 32kg. This is judged against bodyweight and the number of repetitions performed correctly within a 10-minute period. For the biathlon there is a rest period of at least 30 minutes between the two jerk and snatch.

During the one hand events, such as the snatch, the kettlebell is swapped once to the other hand after 5 minutes. For males, the result is taken as the average score and for females it is the total reps.

As an example of the levels of these elite athletes, the current entry level to the WKC Master of Sport World Class Category for a 90kg+ male would be:

- 140 repetitions of the two hand jerk
- 90+ repetitions of the one hand snatch, each side
- 85 repetitions of the two hand clean and jerk.

All of these exercises must be achieved within 10 minutes, using one or two 32kg kettlebells.

Dedication to succeed

In October 2010, Valery Fedorenko completed 70 repetitions with a 60kg kettlebell weight in 9 minutes 15 seconds to set a new world record. This gives the casual kettlebell enthusiast an idea of the dedication required to succeed in the sport of kettlebell lifting.

GLOSSARY

Antagonistic muscles Muscles or muscle groups that perform opposing muscle actions, such as the biceps and triceps, which act as flexors and extensors of the elbow respectively.

Bodyweight drills Exercises that use the weight of the body as resistance, such as pull-ups or press-ups.

Brace To contract the core muscles as a unit to develop intra-abdominal pressure and stabilise the back, hips and pelvis.

Core The muscles that connect the hips and pelvis to the lumbar spine and ribs.

Dead lift The exercise that teaches how to correctly pick up a load from the floor.

Efficiency The ability to perform a task as smoothly and effortlessly as possible, conserving energy and reducing the risk of injury.

Fitness kettlebell Any kettlebell that does not meet the competition standards.

Fixed path machinery A piece of exercise equipment, found in gyms and health clubs, that follows a set path without deviation, commonly referred to as a 'machine' as opposed to freeweight exercises. Examples include seated leg extension and leg curls.

Fluid style The method of kettlebell training used by elite Girevoy to relax and conserve energy.

Force vector The angle that the load is pulled, pressed, lifted or rotated.

Frontal plane stability The ability to avoid any lateral or side-to-side swaying under load, such as lifting a weight on one side or pressing a weight overhead in one hand.

Functional training Exercise that will improve your ability, performance or efficiency in your daily tasks, occupation or sport.

Girevoy kettlebell A kettlebell that meets competition standards and is a standard size across all weights.

Girevoy style (GS) Technique of any person who lifts kettlebells, but today it is a term used to describe the technique of those who compete in kettlebell competitions.

Human movement patterns Movements that humans have performed for thousands of years, and that should be replicated within exercise selection.

Kettlebell Buddy™ A weight that can be screwed onto certain brands of kettlebell to provide an interim increase in weight.

Kettlebell Leash™ A chain that can be screwed onto certain bands of kettlebell to provide an increase in load and to help correct technique.

Kyphosis A prominent rounding of the thoracic spine.

Lactate capacity or power The lactate energy system provides a fast source of energy for exercise. Lactate capacity training improves the size of this energy system, while lactate power training improves the speed at which it can provide energy.

Long cycle A clean is performed between each repetition of the exercise. For example, a long cycle squat is actually a clean and squat.

Lordosis An excessive curvature of the lumbar spine.

Hinging Pivoting or flexing at the hips while maintaining a neutral or flat back position.

Hip rotators The muscles around the hips responsible for hip internal or external rotation.

Pood The traditional kettlebell weight measurement equating to about 16kg.

Progressive resistance A weight that increases throughout the range of the exercise, and commonly includes band resistance or chains. The resistance or load increases as the band tightens or more of the chain is lifted off the ground.

Rack A position where the weight is held on the chest or shoulders.

Remedial drill Any drill used to correct a technique flaw, or biomechanical restriction.

Rigid style A style of kettlebell training where maximal activation of the desired muscles is sought.

Rolfing A system of soft tissue manipulation developed by Ida Rolf, that focuses on releasing myofascial adhesions and improving posture. Also called bodywork manipulation or structural integration.

Rooting Maintaining a strong connection with the floor through the feet.

Rotator cuff The deep muscles around the shoulder responsible for shoulder stability.

Snap The powerful hip extension used in the rigid style of training during any ballistic lift pattern, such as the swing, snatch or clean.

Superset Pairing two exercises together to maximise the amount of work performed in a session or to overload specific muscle groups.

Time-under-tension (TUT) The duration of time that a muscle or group of muscles is under tension for, or put another way, the duration of the set.

VO$_2$max Maximal oxygen consumption – the maximum amount of oxygen that can be inhaled, transported and utilized by the body. It is a gauge of aerobic fitness.

REFERENCES

Bührle, M. and Schmidtbleicher, D. (1981). 'Kompo-. nenten der Maximal- und Schnellkraft.' *Sportwissenschaft.* 11(6):11–27.

Chandler, T.J. & Stone, M.H. (1991). 'The squat exercise in athletic conditioning: A review of the literature.' *National Strength and Conditioning Association Journal* 13 (5).

Farrar, R.E., Mayhew, J.L. & Koch, A.J. (2010). 'Oxygen cost of kettlebell swings.' *The Journal of Strength & Conditioning Research.* 24(4):1034–1036.

Fry, A.C., Kraemer, W.J., Stone, M.H., Warren, B.J., Fleck, S.J., Kearney, J.T. & Gordon, S.E. (1994). 'Endocrine responses to over-reaching before and after 1 year of weightlifting training.' *Canadian Journal of Applied Physiology.* 19(4):400–410.

King, I. (2000). 'Speed of movement. 'http://www.ptonthenet.com/displayarticle.aspx?ArticleID=1022 Accessed in 2007.

Klein, K.K. (1962). 'The knee and the ligaments.' *The Journal of Bone and Joint Surgery.* 44:1191–1193.

Kraemer, W.J., Marchitelli, L., McCurry, D., Mello, R., Dziados, J.E., Harman, E., Frykman, P., Gordon, S.E. & Fleck, S.J. (1990). 'Hormonal and growth factor response to heavy resistance exercise.' *Journal of Applied Physiology.* 69(4):1442–1450.

McGill, S. (2002). *Low Back Disorders.* Human Kinetics (London, UK).

Poliquin, C. (2004). *PICP Theory Manual Level 1.* Poliquin Performance Centre (IL, USA).

Tabata, I., Irisawa, K., Kouzaki, M., Nishimura, K., Ogita, F. & Miyachi, M. (1996). 'Effects of moderate-intensity endurance and high-intensity intermittent training on anaerobic capacity and VO_2max'. *Med Sci Sports Exerc* 28 (10): 1327–30.

Wilson, G.J., Elliott, B.C. & Wood, G.A. (1991). 'The effect on performance of imposing a delay during a stretch-shorten cycle movement.' *Medicine & Science in Sports & Exercise.* 23(3):364–370.

INDEX

acclimatisation 153
adaptation 152
advanced sessions 165–6
alternating bridge press, two kettlebells 134
alternating cleans, two kettlebells 138
alternating swing snatch 73
alternating two hand press, two kettlebells 125, 126
angry cat 35

back squat, one kettlebell in two hands 114
barbell overhead squat 50
beginner sessions 161–2
benefits of training 13–17
bent-over alternating row, two kettlebells 141
bent-over row, one kettlebell and arm support 141
bodyweight side plank 52
bodyweight squat 46, 48–50
bottoms up clean, one kettlebell 138–9
bottoms up rack
    with one hand 25
    with two hands 26
bottoms up snatch
one kettlebell 107
two kettlebells 107–8
bridge press, two kettlebells 133

cardiovascular fitness 13, 15
carrying load pattern 144–7
competitions 4, 5, 19, 167
contraindications 22

core activation 23–4
crossover lunge frontal plane, two kettlebells
    one rack position & one by side 123
    rack position 123
crunch exercise 143–4
crush grip 28

deadlift exercises 99–102
dead position on floor
    in front of body 29
    between legs 29
dead snatch
    from floor, one kettlebell 103–4
    from hang position, one kettlebell 105
    and reverse lunge, one kettlebell 106
    two kettlebells 108
dead swing with finger release, one kettlebell 56
diagonal dead snatch from floor, one kettlebell 106–7
double rack 30
dynamic mobilisation drills 45–7
dynamic resistance training 13

efficiency 18–19
energy, wasting 18
exercise progressions 91–149

farmer's hold 27
farmer's walk, two kettlebells 146
fingertip hold 27
fire hydrant 36

fit bars 12
fitness kettlebells 4–5
flipped clean, one kettlebell 139
flipped rack with one hand see waiter's hold
floor press, two kettlebells 133
fluid style two hand swing 62
forearm strength and endurance 17
foundation exercises 53–90
free weights 13–14
frontal leg swings 47
front squat
    heels elevated, one kettlebell 81–2
    one kettlebell, one hand, flipped grip 113
    one kettlebell and bottoms up grip 111
    one kettlebell in two hands 110
    push press
        one kettlebell 114
        two kettlebells, two hands 114
        two kettlebells, two hands alternating press 115
    two kettlebells in one hand 113
    two kettlebells in two hands 111
    two kettlebells in two hands, heels raised 112
    two kettlebells in two hands, sumo stance 112
functional training 3

gait 148
get up anyhow, two kettlebells 145–6
Girevoy Sport (GS) 3
Girevoy style
    one hand (swing) snatch 73
    two hand rack 31, 91–2
    two hand swing 62
Goldilocks principle 18
good morning 43
    one kettlebell on the back 99

grip
    amount of 19
    strength and endurance 17
    types of 25–31

half snatch 72
hammer curls, one kettlebell 148
hand-to-hand swing, one kettlebell 95
hang position 30
hang snatch, one kettlebell 104–5
hard style two hand swing 62
hip hinge 39
hip rotation 39
history 2–3
human movement patterns 14, 154, 155

inchworm 38
intensity 155–6
intermediate sessions 163–5
International Girya Sport Federation (IGSF) 4
International Union of Kettlebell Lifting (IUKL) 4

kettlebell arm bar 44
kettlebell around the body pass 42
Kettlebell Buddy™ 10
kettlebell figure-of-eight between legs 44
kettlebell halos 43
Kettlebell Leash™ 11
kettlebells 4–12
    anatomy 8–10
    attachments 10–12
    choosing by design 8–10
    history 2–3
    rusting 6
    testing 10
    types of 4–6

weights 6–8
knee to chest 38

lift pattern 14
limited mobility 34
loaded mobilisation drills 42–4
locomotion 148
low-intensity mobilisation drills 35–42
lunge
    frontal plane, two kettlebells, rack position 122
    and overhead reach 45
    and rotation 45
    sagittal plane, two kettlebells, rack position 122

mental focus 17
metabolic acceleration 15
moving/carrying load pattern 144–7
muscle spindles 55

neck mobility 35
neutral spine position 23–4
noise, making 18

one hand assisted dead clean, one kettlebell 75
one hand bent press, one kettlebell 131
one hand dead clean, one kettlebell 75
one hand dead swing 63, 64
one hand front squat 79–82
one hand high pull
    one kettlebell 68
    with release, one kettlebell 109
one hand mini swings, one kettlebell 64
one hand overhead press 82–5
one hand press, one kettlebell
    bottoms up grip 127
    fingertip hold 127
    flipped grip 126

one hand side press, one kettlebell 130
one hand squat press, two kettlebells 134
one hand swing 62–7
    one kettlebell
        and fingers release 96
        and frontal flip 97
        and release at top 96
        and sagittal flip 96
        and a towel 98
        and transverse flip 97
    two kettlebells 98
one hand (swing) clean 73–8
one hand (swing) clean wall drill 78
one hand (swing) snatch 67–73
one hand Turkish get-up 85–8
one hand windmill 88–90
overhead press with rotation, one kettlebell 128
overload 152

periodisation 153–4
pistol grip 25
pistol squat
    one kettlebell
        held in two hands 119
        held in two hands extended 120
        in rack position 118–19
    two kettlebells in rack position 120
plank on two kettlebells with knee raise 149
plateau busters 152
position
    common faults 24
    spinal 23–4
power endurance 15–16
practice 18–19
prayer upward-facing dog 37
preparation exercises 48–52
press pattern 14, 124–36

press-up with kettlebells 135–6
pull pattern 14, 136–41

rack position 74
rack with one hand 25
renegade row, two kettlebells 139–40
repetition maximum (RM) 156
repetitions 156–7
rest periods 159–60
reverse crossover lunge 41
reversibility 153
rigid style two hand swing 62
Romanian deadlift (RDL) 39
    barbell 51
    quad stretch single leg 40
    single leg 40
    two hand swing, one kettlebell 55–6
rotation pattern 142
Russian Kettlebell Certification (RKC) courses 3

safety 20–2
    after training 22
    contraindications 22
    before training 20
    during training 21
sagittal leg swings 47
Sandow, Eugen 2
sciatic nerve mobilisation 41–2
seated rotations, one kettlebell 142
see saw press 125, 126
sets 159
side plank press 135
single arm overhead squat
    one kettlebell 115–16
        and bottoms up or flipped grip 116
    two kettlebells, with deadlift 116
single leg deadlift 101–2
smash pattern 143

snatch variations 103–9
specificity 152–3
Spiderman stretch 36
spinal position 23–4
split dead snatch, one kettlebell 105
split squat
    two kettlebells, rack position 121
    variations 121–2
squat pattern 110–23
squat with one arm overhead, one in rack, two
    kettlebells 117
standard press finish 28
standing crush grip rotation, one kettlebell 142
step and reach 46
step-up with two kettlebells at side 117–18
strength endurance 15–16
strongmen, Victorian 2–3
styles, copying 19
supine bridge 37
supine shuffle, one kettlebell over head 147
supplementary drills 148–9
supplementary movements/exercises 154
swing snatch, two kettlebells 109
swing variations 91–9

tempo 157–9
time-under-tension (TUT) 157, 158
towels 11–12
training
    example sessions 161–6
    principles 152–4
    recommendations 155–60
Tsatsouline, Pavel 3
Turkish get-up
    partial without hand support 144
    with squat, one kettlebell 144–5
two hand anyhow 3, 132
two hand dead clean

from floor, two kettlebells 136–7
　　one kettlebell 75
two hand mini swings, one kettlebell 56–7
two hand overhead squat, two kettlebells 117
two hand power jerk, two kettlebells 129–30
two hand press, two kettlebells 124–5
two hand push press, two kettlebells 128–9
two hand rack 30, 31, 91–2
two hand Romanian deadlift, one kettlebell 100
two hand single leg deadlift, one kettlebell 101–2
two hand split jerk, two kettlebells 129
two hand sumo deadlift, one kettlebell 101
two hand swing 54–62
　　one kettlebell 57–62
　　　　with lateral step 93
　　　　　partner-added push 94
　　　and towel/rope 93–4
　　　style variations 62
two kettlebells 92–3
two hand (swing) clean, two kettlebells 137

upper and lower torso link 16

Victorian strongmen 2–3
volume 159

waiter's bow 39
waiter's hold 26
walk, one kettlebell overhead 147
warm-up 34–47
weights 6–8
World Kettlebell Club (WKC) 4